The Cancer Recovery Plan

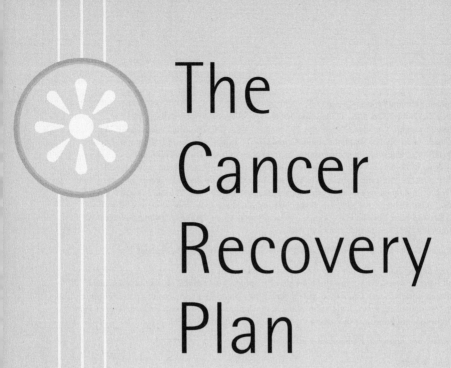

The Cancer Recovery Plan

Maximize Your Cancer
Treatment with This Proven
Nutrition, Exercise, and
Stress-Reduction Program

**D. Barry Boyd, MD,
and Marian Betancourt**

AVERY

A MEMBER OF PENGUIN GROUP (USA) INC. ✳ NEW YORK

Published by the Penguin Group
Penguin Group (USA) Inc., 375 Hudson Street, New York, New York 10014, USA ·
Penguin Group (Canada), 90 Eglinton Avenue East, Suite 700, Toronto, Ontario M4P 2Y3,
Canada (a division of Pearson Penguin Canada Inc.) · Penguin Books Ltd, 80 Strand, London
WC2R 0RL, England · Penguin Ireland, 25 St Stephen's Green, Dublin 2, Ireland (a division
of Penguin Books Ltd) · Penguin Group (Australia), 250 Camberwell Road, Camberwell,
Victoria 3124, Australia (a division of Pearson Australia Group Pty Ltd) · Penguin Books India
Pvt Ltd, 11 Community Centre, Panchsheel Park, New Delhi–110 017, India · Penguin Group
(NZ), Cnr Airborne and Rosedale Roads, Albany, Auckland 1310, New Zealand (a division
of Pearson New Zealand Ltd) · Penguin Books (South Africa) (Pty) Ltd, 24 Sturdee Avenue,
Rosebank, Johannesburg 2196, South Africa

Penguin Books Ltd, Registered Offices: 80 Strand, London WC2R 0RL, England

Library of Congress Cataloging-in-Publication Data

Boyd, D. Barry.
    The cancer recovery plan / D. Barry Boyd and Marian Betancourt.
        p.   cm.
    Includes bibliographical references and index.
    ISBN 1-58333-230-8
        1. Cancer—Nutritional aspects.   2. Cancer—Popular works.   3. Stress management.
    4. Physical fitness.   5. Weight loss.   I. Betancourt, Marian.   II. Title.
    RC268.45.B69   2005   2005041220
    616.99'40654—dc22

Printed in the United States of America
10 9 8 7 6 5 4 3 2

Book design by Lovedog Studio

Most Avery books are available at special quantity discounts for bulk purchases for sales promo-
tions, premiums, fund-raising, and educational needs. Special books or book excerpts also can
be created to fit specific needs. For details, write Penguin Group (USA) Inc. Special Markets,
375 Hudson Street, New York, NY 10014.

This book is dedicated to my patients. It is their
journey that has both inspired and driven me to seek the
answers that have led to the ideas in this book.

—DBB

This is also in memory of Priscilla Dahl.

—MB

Contents

Acknowledgments

I AM INDEBTED TO many individuals for their research and teaching, but for reasons of brevity, many who are appreciated must go unacknowledged. I particularly want to thank those physicians whose work or research has inspired me, and those who have taken an interest in my work and clinical care: Myron Winick, Richard Rivlin, Daniel Nixon, Herbert Yu, David Felten, Mary Maida, Susan Maynes, David Yee, Joy Craddock, Dwight McKee, Herbert Benson, Bernadette Johnson, Guruchuran S. Khalsa, Peggy Huddleston, James Gordon, Michael Lerner, and Woodson Merrell.

I also want to thank my coauthor, Marian Betancourt, and our agent, Vicky Bijur, who put up with frequent delays and the inevitable conflicts of a practicing physician.

I am indebted to my staff at Integrative Oncology and to the nurses and assistants on "Med-3" and the Greenwich Hospital library staff, who were always there to assist me in my research. I especially want to thank my wife, Robin, and my children, Erica, Anthony, Brendan, and Dylan. Without their presence and support, neither my work nor this book would have been possible.

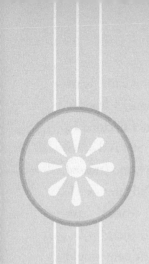

Introduction

CANCER—A SCARY DIAGNOSIS, INDEED. Once doctors utter that dreaded word, most people tend to put their care solely in their doctors' hands and pray that the chemotherapy, radiation, and/or surgery these professionals prescribe will cure them. Others spurn medical care altogether, turning instead to unproven and potentially dangerous alternative treatments. In addition to the best medical care possible, nutrition, exercise, and stress reduction are absolutely necessary to make your cancer treatment more effective and prevent cancer's return. My aim is to help you become a more informed patient—one who will take an active role in your cancer treatment and future well-being. Throughout this book, you'll read stories of my patients who have benefited from this kind of care. Some came to me after leaving other doctors who had given them a hopeless prognosis.

My integrative oncology practice evolved from my early years studying the biochemistry of nutrition. It wasn't until I learned about how nutrition affects health and disease that I decided to study medicine and then oncology. Long before the public and other doctors acknowledged that being overweight, sedentary, and stressed are related to cancer, I was researching these links, and later developed a medical practice based on this knowledge. I worked with my patients to control their weight and encouraged them to become physically active because I knew that their treatment would be more effective, giving them a much better prognosis. I firmly believe—and have seen the results—that the best conventional medical care must be combined with integrative therapy. Nutrition, exercise, and state of mind are critical to cancer treatment.

As we all know by now, Americans are dangerously overweight because they eat too much and don't work off that excess energy with physical activity. Most people do understand now that this is probably a factor in diabetes and heart disease, but few see the link to cancer. The result of too much food and not enough exercise is insulin resistance. This leads to an imbalance in the hormonal dynamics of your body that affects all the cells in your body. It especially sets you up for the type of uncontrolled cell proliferation that leads to cancer. This condition also interferes with chemotherapy and other cancer treatment, as well—and it can be *caused* by some cancer treatments and the stress of having cancer.

Insulin resistance is the primary component of the metabolic syndrome (also known as syndrome X). It is essentially a biological imbalance caused by too much food, too much stress, and too little physical activity. It is characteristic of many advanced cancers and is also a cause, especially of hormonal cancers such as breast, uterine, and prostate. It is also linked with digestive cancers, such as colon, pancreatic, and esophageal, as well as liver and kidney cancer. In other words, the cancers of civilization—those that reflect our lifestyle—are rising in tandem with the number of people who are overweight. Forty percent of people over forty have the metabolic syndrome, which means that 40 percent of cancer patients over forty also have it, though I suspect its prevalence is much higher among cancer patients.

Some doctors are beginning to recognize this relationship between cancer and the metabolic syndrome, but most are still unaware, and all of them have virtually ignored it as a risk factor in the progression of cancer—or in successful treatment.

Most cancer researchers have been focused on the immune system. Much research has been done to find cancer cures through the immune system. As a result, much of the lay public, too, believes they must strengthen their immune system to prevent or fight cancer. Some are so concerned that, if diagnosed with cancer, they won't even get conventional treatment like chemotherapy, for fear it will damage their immune system. Others take unproven and expensive nutritional supplements, thinking they will offer protection. Without seeking medical advice, they often sabotage their treatment with these supplements. But we have been looking in the wrong place. It is the endocrine system, with its glands and hormones, that is the real culprit in most cancers.

This book will help you understand why the metabolic syndrome is a key player in cancer and cancer treatment. You'll learn how to work with your doctors to identify this syndrome if you have it—and how it affects your treatment. You will learn how to diversify your diet, increase physical activity, reduce stress—and thus, your insulin levels—and reduce the side effects of cancer and its treatment. My program takes into account the whole person, not just the cancer patient. For most people, it's the beginning of a changed lifestyle that helps them remain cancer free and healthier for the rest of their lives.

Controlling weight, getting active, and reducing stress are not simply nuances of basic well-being; they are absolutely necessary to the successful treatment of cancer. In addition to the best medical care, a cancer patient needs to take a three-pronged approach to total care:

1. Control weight with a sensible nutrition plan.
2. Get physically active.
3. Reduce stress.

Unless all three of these areas are addressed with integrative therapies, cancer treatment can be sabotaged.

Like many oncologists, I have patients with many different cancers who have defied the odds. Hundreds of patients with advanced cancer came to me with discouraging prognoses after conventional cancer treatment, and they are here today to tell their stories throughout this book. Some have no evidence of the advanced cancer they were originally treated for. Others remain in a symbiotic relationship with their disease, living high-quality lives while receiving therapy as needed to maintain control.

Cancer is not a hopeless disease.

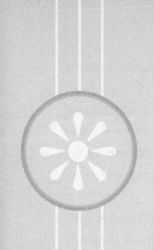

CHAPTER 1

The Missing Link: What You Need to Know about Cancer Treatment and the Metabolic Syndrome

MORE DIE IN THE United States of too much food than of too little." John Kenneth Galbraith wrote that in his 1958 book, *The Affluent Society*. Today we are finally beginning to acknowledge how right he was. The rising numbers of cancer cases over the last fifty years are typically cancers of civilization, disease of affluence.

In early 2003, the American Cancer Society published their nearly twenty-year study of more than 900,000 men and women, one of the largest and longest-duration studies of its kind, which demonstrated a significant increase in death from almost all cancers in people who are overweight or obese. An unexpectedly broad spectrum of cancers is involved, including hormonal cancers such as breast and endometrial, as well as nonhormonal cancers such as colon, pancreatic, and liver. It even included the blood malignancies lymphoma and myeloma. Only a few cancers were found to have no link to excess weight.

The study gained wide attention among cancer researchers as well as the general public. Ironically, just as this new and compelling association has been noted, we are simultaneously being warned of the growing epidemic of obesity within our population, often beginning in early childhood.

The more we understand obesity, the more we realize that simply being overweight and inactive—in other words, living the modern American lifestyle—produces basic hormonal and metabolic changes that make it easier for cancer to gain a foothold. And once it has a foothold, these same dynamics make cancer more difficult to treat and potentially cure. Cancer treatment itself often causes weight gain and the metabolic syndrome.

For many years, being overweight was viewed simply as a cosmetic problem, to be hidden behind designer clothing or lost with the latest fad diet. But, of course, obesity is now known to be a major health problem. Fat is metabolically and hormonally active tissue. Fat cells behave like endocrine cells, constantly producing and secreting a wide variety of hormones and other so-called growth factors or cytokines into the bloodstream. (We'll explain these later.) Normally, these natural body chemicals carry out many necessary functions, such as regulating the metabolism of fats and carbohydrates, affecting overall energy balance, and encouraging cells to grow and divide in a precise and regulated way. But excess body fat causes greater amounts of these hormones and growth factors to be continually pumped into the bloodstream. As a result, an overweight person's cells are urged to grow and divide at an accelerated rate. When cell division and replication occurs more frequently, the chances increase that something could go wrong in the process. One such possibility is the kind of random mutation that can lead to cancer.

The Nature of Cancer

Cancer is a multistep process. Initially there are mutations in critical genes, followed by progressive accumulation of further genetic changes that lead to precancerous changes, then to early in situ (meaning in one place) cancer followed by truly invasive cancers. Over time, these invasive cancers acquire more changes, become more aggressive, and travel to other organs. This is metastasis.

Insulin and other growth chemicals in the body enhance the proliferation of tumor cells, making more cells vulnerable to these genetic changes. This hastens the speed of progression to a more malignant state. So, tissues with an inherently low rate of cell replication, such as brain and bone, have a much lower rate of cancers in general than rapidly reproducing tissues in the colon and breast.

There are two ways to avoid this cellular progression, and thus avoid cancer. One is to avoid mutagens, but this is beyond our control because many are in water, food, or cosmic radiation. The other way is to reduce your exposure to tumor promoters, such as visceral abdominal fat and related insulin and insulin growth factors. This you can control with diet, exercise, and stress reduction. (Visceral fat is hidden among abdominal organs and is different from subcutaneous fat located just beneath the skin. Many people of normal weight have visceral fat.)

The Common Link

According to the 2003 American Cancer Society study, there is a direct relationship between the amount of excess weight and the risk of death from most cancers. In other words, the higher the body mass index (BMI), a measure of weight in relation to height, the greater the risk of cancer death. (See chapter 2 for more about BMI.)

We hope this new information will spur physicians to provide exercise and dietary advice to their patients (the American Association of Gastroenterologists has already urged members to do this) and influence the insurance industry to increase reimbursement for this essential component of health care.

You may carry a risk factor for cancer because of age or sex or even family history, but if you reduce the risk factors in your control, you lower your risk dramatically. If you already have cancer, you can increase your chance of survival in the same way—by reducing lifestyle factors that are making your cancer more aggressive.

The Metabolic Syndrome

The metabolic syndrome is a cluster of conditions that includes high levels of blood sugar and cholesterol, high blood pressure, inflammation, and abdominal obesity, which together greatly increase the risk of adult-onset diabetes, heart disease, and cancer. The presence of any of these three conditions would mean you may have the syndrome, which is usually—but not always—the result of poor diet, lack of exercise, and unremitting stress. It's also sometimes caused by cancer, but we'll get to that later. Fat cells spew hormones and inflammatory cells that lead to a chain of events that cause the metabolic syndrome and set you up for cancer. The metabolic syndrome is increasing among adults in the United States, especially in women with a large waist circumference, high blood pressure, and high triglycerides.

Chronic Low-Grade Inflammation

Until recently, the importance of chronic low-grade inflammation in the metabolic syndrome was not well understood, so it warrants some explanation here. (The other characteristics of the metabolic syndrome, such as abdominal obesity and high sugar and cholesterol levels, are more easily understood.)

The presence of systemic, chronic low-grade inflammation may foster the proliferation of abnormal cells and facilitate their transformation to cancer. In other words, it may be the engine that drives many of the cancers of middle and old age as well as heart disease, Alzheimer's, and other diseases.

Inflammation stimulates tumor cells to proliferate; it increases the growth of blood vessels that feed the cancer cells. Chronic inflammation adversely affects survival in many cancers (colon, breast, esophageal, pancreatic, renal cell, head and neck, ovarian, lung, myeloma, and non-Hodgkin's lymphoma) as well as advanced cancer in general. In most studies, the impact of the inflammatory state on prognosis was independent of stage (progression of the disease) and grade (speed of cell proliferation) of cancer and the presence of other disease conditions.

Here's how inflammation occurs. Whenever your body is hurt, a series of events is triggered. When you cut your finger, specialized sentinel cells stationed throughout your body alert your immune system that bacteria may be present. Some of those cells, called mast cells, release histamine. This makes nearby small blood vessels (capillaries) leaky, so that small amounts of plasma can pour out and slow down the invading bacteria. At the same time, other faraway immune defenders enter the battle, while macrophages, another group of sentinels, begin an immediate counterattack by releasing cytokines. These chemicals signal for reinforcements. Soon, your injured finger is flooded with immune cells that destroy pathogens and damaged tissue alike. In this war, both sides are wiped out. In the disease state, this kind of inflammation becomes chronic. The strategies our bodies used for early survival are obsolete and may even be turning against us. We are living longer now and those same inflammatory strategies may slip beyond our control.

Many of the attributes of a Western lifestyle, such as a diet high in sugars and saturated fats, accompanied by little or no exercise, make it easier for the body to become inflamed—and stay inflamed. Fat cells behave a lot like immune cells, spewing out inflammatory cytokines, particularly as you gain weight. Cells known as macrophages also infiltrate adipose tissue, further increasing the cytokine burden. Thus, there is a complex interplay between inflammation, insulin, and fat. Losing weight induces those fat cells to produce fewer cytokines. So does thirty minutes a day of regular exercise.

Depression, which is common in the cancer patient, has also been linked to increasing inflammatory cytokines. Some of the most severe responses to stress include a sense of hopelessness and helplessness, loss of appetite, impaired sleep, loss of interest in pleasurable activities, and withdrawal from friends. The body responds by altering the production of hormones, including insulin, and raising some cytokine levels typical of inflammation. Thus, it's conceivable that severe stress has a very definite impact on cancer outcomes.

A *Time* magazine cover story in February 2004 reported that doctors and drug makers were finally putting inflammation at the top of their research and development list. One drug maker said his company's *entire* research and development effort is now focused on inflammation and cancer. Just a few years ago nobody was interested in this idea; now, not only are other oncologists discussing this concept with me, so are cardiologists, rheumatologists, allergists, and neurologists.

I will show you how to test for the inflammatory state in chapter 2.

The Endocrine System

In order to know how the metabolic syndrome develops, let's look at the endocrine system. It is made up of glands that produce and secrete hormones that regulate your body's growth, metabolism (the physical and chemical processes of the body), and sexual development and function. The hormones that may lead to the onset of the metabolic syndrome are insulin, growth hormones, and the stress hormones epinephrine and cortisol.

The body creates hormones to act as chemical messengers to transfer information from one set of cells to another to coordinate the functions of different parts of the body. The major glands of this system are the hypothalamus, pituitary, thyroid, parathyroids, adrenals, pineal body, and the reproductive organs (ovaries and testes). The pancreas is also involved in hormone production as well as in digestion.

Insulin

Insulin is a hormone that works with other hormones in your body, including sex, growth, and stress hormones. It regulates blood sugar levels and fat metabolism. The carbohydrates you ingest are broken down into glucose and transported into the bloodstream. Insulin is secreted by the pancreas in response to rising sugar levels. It then allows the blood sugar to be transported across cell membranes in a variety of cells, such as muscle and liver, to provide glucose as fuel for a few hours. When glucose remains unavailable as fuel, as happens with prolonged fasting or starvation, insulin production is switched off and the body burns its own fat as fuel. When abundant glucose is available, the body, in the presence of continued insulin secretion, will add to the fat stores to provide fuel for "a rainy day." Throughout most of human evolution, food supplies were unpredictable and it was necessary to have a mechanism to store those extra calories in times of plenty. This trait becomes problematic when we have abundant year-round, calorie-dense foods that don't require expending much effort to obtain (chasing and catching that gazelle or rummaging in the soil for edible tuberous plant foods).

When insulin levels remain low, you will burn your own fat and keep your weight down. However, when they are persistently elevated, you won't burn off fat but will add to those stores with insulin's help. This is what is happening to more and more people who consume more calories than they burn.

Insulin Resistance

The more overweight you are, the more insulin your pancreas will pump out when you eat, and the more likely you are to develop insulin resistance, the fundamental abnormality in the metabolic syndrome. In effect, your cells become less and less sensitive to the action of the insulin, and so your pancreas needs to generate ever greater amounts to maintain a normal blood sugar level. Thus, as you progressively gain weight, insulin makes it easier to store fat and harder to lose it.

Not all stored fat is created equal, however. It has become clear that the typical middle-aged paunch, usually a sign of fat surrounding our organs (visceral fat), is particularly linked to increasing insulin resistance typical of the metabolic syndrome. We recognize it by our increasing belt size or waist circumference. By middle age, over a quarter of the population has this condition. And since most people get cancer in middle age, many of them will have the metabolic syndrome.

Under normal conditions, hormones simply carry out basic life functions, such as encouraging cells to grow and divide in a precise and regulated way. When cells divide and grow more frequently, as they do with increased insulin levels due to resistance, there's more chance something could go wrong in the process. For example, the lining of the colon may be particularly sensitive to the effects of insulin because it is composed of cells that already divide at a rapid rate. In a healthy body there is hormonal balance involving insulin, insulin-like growth factors, sex, and stress hormones.

Insulin resistance may develop with cancer treatment related to weight gain (you'll find out more about this in chapter 3).

Growth Hormones

Insulin-like growth factors are proteins produced by the liver and other cells that bind to receptors on the cell surface and activate cellular proliferation. IGF-1, the most abundant of this family of growth factors, promotes the proliferation of many cell types and is particularly important in the early stage of growth and development. IGF-1 is a powerful growth factor for many cancer cell types.

While IGF and insulin are related, they are not the same and are regulated differently in the body. However, in states of prolonged high insulin that are typical of the metabolic syndrome (and overweight), the liver production of some of the binding proteins circulating in the blood will be suppressed. When the binding protein is suppressed, more of the growth factor circulates in a free unbound state, leading to higher levels of exposure to cells, both normal and malignant. Thus, cells—including cancer cells—are stimulated to grow.

No malignancy better illustrates the complex effects of insulin and insulin growth factors in combination with other hormones on tumor development, as well as outcome, than breast cancer. This reflects in part the extensive research devoted to this disease because of the political action of women and the resulting understanding of these complexities. While the importance of estrogen in breast cancer development and outcome has been long appreciated, particularly in postmenopausal women with hormone-sensitive breast tumors, the impact of high insulin levels is increasingly recognized as playing an important role both in development and outcome.

Sex Hormones

Sex hormones are steroids produced and secreted by the ovaries in women and the prostate gland in men. These chemicals orchestrate many biological activities beginning shortly after conception by determining whether the developing fetus is male or female. The primary female sex hormones are estrogen and progesterone. Male sex hormones are called androgens. Testosterone is the primary androgen.

In all women, the ovaries stop producing estrogen after menopause, but body fat is an estrogen pump and continues to produce low levels of the hormone. Studies on overweight postmenopausal women reveal higher levels of circulating estrogen than in women at or near ideal weight.

Too much estrogen can cause breast cancer. It is widely believed that overweight postmenopausal women experience higher cancer risk because their larger fat deposits continue to pump relatively high amounts of estrogen into the bloodstream. Because body fat produces a wide range of hormones and hormonelike substances, some scientists predict that excess body fat will ultimately prove to be most strongly implicated in the development of the hormonal cancers. Because much of this estrogen effect develops over years or decades, it takes many years before it causes trouble.

Testosterone, the major male hormone, is not quite like estrogen in that it is not produced by fat cells. Nevertheless, it plays a similar role in prostate cancer. This cancer is a disease of aging in men and it develops from long-term exposure to testosterone.

Stress Hormones

Stress prompts the body to produce cortisol—the stress hormone—which in turn adds to abdominal fat, such as a potbelly or love handles. Cortisol, a steroid hormone, controls how the body uses fat, protein, carbohydrates, and minerals and helps reduce inflammation. Body fat tends to settle more quickly into the abdominal area, so high levels of cortisol increase the abdominal fat stores.

Even in someone of moderate weight, this fat is associated with the production of higher levels of insulin than fat found elsewhere in the body. Cancer treatment itself raises your stress level, which, in turn, leads to higher cortisol and increased abdominal fat. Among the general public and cancer patients and their families, there is a commonly held belief that cancer is closely linked to stress. Yet most physicians view this association as tenuous at best. And while most people view stress as an important association, they failed to make the connection of stress and abdominal body fat.

Acute stress occurs when a single event, like being in a burning building, sets off an alarm response in the brain. The adrenal glands get the stress signal and release a cascade of stress hormones. With prolonged stress, such as being in a war or living with cancer and its treatment, stress hormones become chronically elevated. They ramp up anxiety centers in the brain, causing more signals to flow to the adrenal glands, releasing more stress hormones. The system sets up a vicious cycle.

It is well known that cortisol is linked to insulin resistance. Cushing's syndrome, a hormonal disorder caused by the body's exposure to high levels of cortisol, is characterized by visceral obesity and insulin resistance. Similarly, infusions of cortisol in levels seen in severe stress will result in impaired insulin sensitivity. In animal studies, chronic stress resulted in increased cortisol levels, increased insulin levels, and weight gain, unrelated to how many calories the animals consumed or burned off with exercise.

Who Has the Metabolic Syndrome?

The American Institute for Cancer Research found that the metabolic syndrome is present in over 20 percent of the adult United States population and in 40 percent of people over forty. Unfortunately it may be unequally distributed in the population. The syndrome was highest in Mexican Americans and lowest in black Americans of both sexes. Risk is also growing in the Asian population, where obesity is rising rapidly. Women are at higher risk for metabolic syndrome at a lower weight. The reasons for these differences are not well understood. The metabolic syndrome seems to increase with higher body mass index, advancing age, current smoking, high carbohydrate intake, low household income, no alcohol consumption, and physical *inactivity*, as well as genetic familial predisposition.

Malnutrition in the first year of life also increases the risk of insulin resistance and glucose intolerance in early adulthood. It is accompanied by rapid weight gain in adolescence. Again, it goes back to evolution. If fetuses are constantly deprived of calories during prenatal development, the presumption is that their metabolic state will be permanently altered to enhance energy storage (fat production). When food is around, those people will produce body fat more aggressively.

And last but certainly not least, many cancer patients develop the metabolic syndrome.

How Cancer Treatment Causes the Metabolic Syndrome

Chemotherapy treatment can bring on the metabolic syndrome. And this is critical to know for treatment as well as follow-up care to avoid recurrence of cancer or a new illness. Many doctors don't bother to counsel their patients after treatment. Once cancer treatment is completed, most patients are left on their own to cope with the rest of their lives. This is what I call falling off the cliff. While the cancer physician may check their blood periodically in the next few months following treatment for signs of cancer, few (if any) monitor their patients' metabolic profile, including weight gain, nutrition, exercise, and stress reduction. Patients are left in free fall. That's why I teach my patients to continue the programs they learned in my office during treatment. I know cancer and its treatment cause a variety of changes in their bodies that can increase their chance of a recurrence or even of another cancer: weight gain or loss, postchemotherapy fatigue, and other conditions can last for years. Conditions that result from treatment need to be taken care of during treatment and *treated for the rest of your life* to assure a good quality of life. This is why you need integrative cancer therapy.

Why You Need Integrative Cancer Therapy

Cancer patients feel a genuine need to take control of their care. They need a program with good conventional medicine that also empowers them to do something for themselves—like learning how better nutrition, exercise, and stress reduction aid their treatment. More important, this kind of medicine gives the doctor an opportunity to embrace the potential for self-care that so many patients undertake and provide them with a safe and effective means of both treating cancer and ensuring good health and a long life.

The purpose of integrative care is to mesh the best of conventional medical care with the best and most appropriate complementary therapy. That is, to see that your body and mind are functioning at their best during your cancer treatment and after.

This is total therapy and its purpose is to give the best possible way for you to overcome cancer, prevent its return, and return to full health. While an increasing number of physicians use integrative techniques, it is often a hit-and-miss approach. The insulin-cancer relationship provides a sound scientific basis for many integrative cancer therapies, including nutrition and exercise and stress reduction. This is increasingly important because the use of mind-body approaches is still dismissed by most conventional physicians who do not appreciate the potential biological basis on which these approaches work and thus don't consider it an important adjunct to conventional cancer therapy.

Once your metabolic profile is determined, you will have a better sense of how treatment will affect you and what other steps to take during and after treatment. Even if you are not insulin resistant, that may change during treatment. Our integrative therapy always includes specific medical treatment for the cancer, treatment to prevent weight gain (or loss) and insulin resistance, treatment for side effects, and a plan for long-term health to avoid cancer recurrence.

How a Misconception about the Immune System Can Sabotage Treatment

For years, science has been looking at the immune system for ways to eliminate disease, including cancer. I want to emphasize here that it is the endocrine system we need to be looking at in cancer treatment.

Because of this widely held misconception about the role of the immune system and cancer, patients are driven unwittingly to sabotage their own cancer treatment. Many mistakenly avoid any conventional therapy because of their known immunosuppressive effects and thus, the fear of enhancing rather than controlling tumor progression.

Chemotherapy, for example, does compromise the immune system because it destroys many cells, not just cancer cells. In addition, many patients try alternative therapies along with their medical therapy, hoping they will improve their immune function and improve their response to treatments or repair the damage the treatments produce. These, again, are based on unproven assumptions.

In addition, much of the work in mind-body medicine, including meditation, guided imagery, and cancer support groups, has focused on the effect on the immune system as an explanation for their potential benefits. By continuing to emphasize this connection, we fail to recognize the biochemical response in the endocrine system, clearly of greater importance in protecting patients against the progression of cancer. Despite hundreds of scientific studies linking insulin to cancer's cause and progression, remarkably few doctors have yet to appreciate this connection. This is like not seeing the forest for the trees. Doctors have known this for years but never paid attention to it as a target for treatment.

Some doctors are beginning to recognize this relationship between cancer and the metabolic syndrome, the biological imbalance caused by too much food, too much stress, and too little physical activity. But most are still unaware, and all of them have virtually ignored it as a risk factor in the progression of cancer— *or its impact on successful treatment*. When cancer patients lose weight during treatment, or feel too nauseated to eat, doctors may be more inclined to urge them to eat anything at all. Doctors are understandably reluctant to urge sick and weak patients to get some exercise, but there are ways it can be done gently and gradually.

My goal is making people understand that losing weight, becoming active, and reducing stress are not simply nuances of basic well-being. They are absolutely necessary to the successful treatment of cancer. I believe that, in addition to the best medical care, a cancer patient needs to take a three-pronged approach to total care. And unless all three of these areas are addressed—nutrition, exercise, and stress reduction—cancer treatment can be sabotaged.

The Critical Triad: Nutrition, Exercise, Stress Reduction

The metabolic syndrome must be considered as a crucial target during the treatment of cancer. The triad of nutrition, exercise, and stress reduction form the foundation of this approach. Integrative practitioners have long emphasized these lifestyle dynamics and the insulin-cancer hypothesis validates these interventions in the care of every cancer patient. You should be provided with options for both conventional and integrative approaches that are individualized for your needs.

* **Control weight with a sensible nutrition plan.** The public is confused by contradictory studies that attempt to isolate particular foods or nutrients in reducing cancer risk. There is no single cancer prevention food that is crucial. An entire new understanding is coming to the surface that it is how nutrition and exercise affect weight and insulin that is most crucial and not simply particular nutrients. (Later in the book, you'll learn specifics about how nutrition and a dietary plan can help your cancer prognosis.)
* **Get physically active.** Moderate activity, such as daily walking, will not only fight the fatigue from cancer treatment but will limit the increase of insulin levels, thus making your chemotherapy or hormone therapy more effective.
* **Reduce stress.** The central role of stress reduction is crucial, particularly given evidence that ongoing severe stress can lead to abdominal obesity and insulin resistance in

the face of diet and activity levels that would otherwise be protective.

All patients are individuals, physically and emotionally as well as in their cancer treatment and how it affects them. All of this is taken into account when planning for treatment. First, I respect the importance of good conventional medicine and never do anything that would interfere with that. But that therapy needs to be enhanced so my patients have a better chance at curing their cancer and preventing its return.

My program is about healthy living. That's what this book is all about.

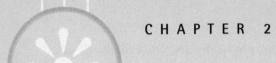

CHAPTER 2

Find Out Your Metabolic Profile

DO YOU KNOW YOUR body mass index? What about your waist-hip ratio? Do you know if you have high levels of insulin in your blood? And what is your mental adjustment to cancer? Most people do not know these things. And doctors, unless they are endocrinologists, don't routinely check patients—even cancer patients—for these factors. You will need to talk with your doctor about this and ask for a metabolic assessment.

If you are like the majority of cancer patients, you are being treated by an oncologist, a surgeon, a radiologist, and other specialists. In addition, your primary-care physician has a role in your care. This is the way it should be because you need the best possible medical care you can get. However, this care by committee may be leaving out the type of overall care you need. Your doctor may give you the best surgery, radiation, or chemotherapy for your cancer but make no suggestions about your lifestyle or general health. Is he or she concerned that you are overweight or have a spare tire around your middle? That you are a couch potato? That the stress of having cancer is an added biological burden?

Many patients are left with little guidance from their doctors. In fact, doctors often shortchange patients when they ask about diet and exercise or stress reduction, because of a busy medical practice or limited knowledge. While they may tell their patients that these lifestyle considerations are important for cardiovascular health, they often don't believe they have any significant effect on cancer cause or treatment. This is frustrating to patients who want such guidance. Today's patients are more knowledgeable about health and willing to discuss new ideas with their doctors.

In my practice, we do an individual metabolic profile for all of our cancer patients, whether or not they appear to have the metabolic syndrome. This includes vital signs such as blood pressure and temperature, a physical assessment with body mass index (BMI), waist circumference and waist-hip ratio, and body fat composition. If hidden internal fat (visceral) is suspected, then a CT scan or abdominal ultrasound is sometimes done to determine if it is present. While a CT scan is routine for anyone with metastatic cancer in order to diagnose and determine the stage of the disease, doctors rarely use it to evaluate the body fat. However, simple measures of BMI and waist size are easy and reliable in most patients.

Each patient's health history, along with current information about cancer surgery and treatment, is evaluated. (We also delve deeply into their diet history; you'll learn more about this in chapter 5.) Your early health history is vital, especially about what happened between your adolescent and adult years. For example if you gained ten to fifteen pounds during those years, this alerts us to look for the metabolic syndrome. Another indicator would be a rapid weight gain in the year prior to the cancer diagnosis. This gain is not your fault, but it may be associated with a more aggressive cancer. By knowing this, we can treat you more effectively and protect you after treatment.

A variety of blood tests is also performed, and you'll find more about these below.

Last but not least, a psychological profile should be done to measure the effect of stress on your treatment and your emotional response to cancer and treatment. This provides your doctors with a baseline for appropriate stress reduction and psychological interventions.

About 35 percent of my patients have the metabolic syndrome and hypertension is fairly common. Very few oncologists will routinely give these tests to cancer patients—*so you need to ask for them*. They are critical to a truly integrative care program.

The Physical Assessment

When I meet a cancer patient, I can see obvious excessive weight, but often thinner people have hidden fat that I cannot see. Someone with a normal BMI of 20 to 27 may have insulin resistance and be metabolically obese, although this is less common. Even a minimal elevation of weight may show early signs of insulin resistance. On the other hand, some overweight people are metabolically normal, so it's important to test for indications of metabolic syndrome before jumping to conclusions.

Anyone can have the metabolic syndrome but it is most often found in those who are overweight. For example, fewer than 10 percent of people with a healthy body weight have the syndrome, compared with 40 to 50 percent of those with a BMI greater than 35.

People with prominent weight in their abdominal area (visceral fat) are more likely to develop the metabolic syndrome than people with the same amount of body weight more evenly distributed.

Waist circumference is a good predictor and is one of the diagnostic criteria for the metabolic syndrome.

If you have the metabolic syndrome, then you have high fasting sugar levels, triglycerides over 150, blood pressure greater than 130 over 85, waist circumference greater than 40 in men and 35 in women, and level of good cholesterol (HDL) under 40. Any three of these measures would identify a majority of people with metabolic syndrome. We may do a skin-fold measure—simply to check the amount of fat in the underarm area—but this is not routine.

Calculate Your Body Mass Index (BMI)

The BMI measure is a formula that considers weight and height to determine whether you have excessive body fat. If you weigh 173 pounds and you are five feet four, you have a body mass index of 30. That means you are obese.

If Your BMI is . . .	You are . . .
Less than 18	Underweight
18.5–24.9	Normal
25–29.9	Overweight
30 or above	Obese

There is a complicated mathematical formula for calculating your BMI, but you can do it the easy way by looking at the chart on page 26. There are also many Web sites where you can simply key in your height and weight and your BMI will be calculated instantly. One such site is maintained by the National Institutes of Health at www.nhlbisupport.com/bmi/bmicalc.htm.

Body Mass Index Table

	Normal						Overweight					Obese						
BMI	19	20	21	22	23	24	25	26	27	28	29	30	31	32	33	34	35	36

Height (inches)

BODY WEIGHT (POUNDS)

Height	19	20	21	22	23	24	25	26	27	28	29	30	31	32	33	34	35	36
58	91	96	100	105	110	115	119	124	129	134	138	143	148	153	158	162	167	172
59	94	99	104	109	114	119	124	128	133	138	143	148	153	158	163	168	173	178
60	97	102	107	112	118	123	128	133	138	143	148	153	158	163	168	174	179	184
61	100	106	111	116	122	127	132	137	143	148	153	158	164	169	174	180	185	190
62	104	109	115	120	126	131	136	142	147	153	158	164	169	175	180	186	191	196
63	107	113	118	124	130	135	141	146	152	158	163	169	175	180	186	191	197	203
64	110	116	122	128	134	140	145	151	157	163	169	174	180	186	192	197	204	209
65	114	120	126	132	138	144	150	156	162	168	174	180	186	192	198	204	210	216
66	118	124	130	136	142	148	155	161	167	173	179	186	192	198	204	210	216	223
67	121	127	134	140	146	153	159	166	172	178	185	191	198	204	211	217	223	230
68	125	131	138	144	151	158	164	171	177	184	190	197	203	210	216	223	230	236
69	128	135	142	149	155	162	169	176	182	189	196	203	209	216	223	230	236	243
70	132	139	146	153	160	167	174	181	188	195	202	209	216	222	229	236	243	250
71	136	143	150	157	165	172	179	186	193	200	208	215	222	229	236	243	250	257
72	140	147	154	162	169	177	184	191	199	206	213	221	228	235	242	250	258	265
73	144	151	159	166	174	182	189	197	204	212	219	227	235	242	250	257	265	272
74	148	155	163	171	179	186	194	202	210	218	225	233	241	249	256	264	272	280
75	152	160	168	176	184	192	200	208	216	224	232	240	248	256	264	272	279	287
76	156	164	172	180	189	197	205	213	221	230	238	246	254	263	271	279	287	295

Source: Adapted from *Clinical Guidelines on the Identification, Evaluation, and Treatment of Overweight and Obesity in Adults: The Evidence Report.*

| Obese | | | Extreme Obesity | | | | | | | | | | | | | | |
37	38	39	40	41	42	43	44	45	46	47	48	49	50	51	52	53	54

BODY   WEIGHT   (POUNDS)

37	38	39	40	41	42	43	44	45	46	47	48	49	50	51	52	53	54
177	181	186	191	196	201	205	210	215	220	224	229	234	239	244	248	253	258
183	188	193	198	203	208	212	217	222	227	232	237	242	247	252	257	262	267
189	194	199	204	209	215	220	225	230	235	240	245	250	255	261	266	271	276
195	201	206	211	217	222	227	232	238	243	248	254	259	264	269	275	280	285
202	207	213	218	224	229	235	240	246	251	256	262	267	273	278	284	289	295
208	214	220	225	231	237	242	248	254	259	265	270	278	282	287	293	299	304
215	221	227	232	238	244	250	256	262	267	273	279	285	291	296	302	308	314
222	228	234	240	246	252	258	264	270	276	282	288	294	300	306	312	318	324
229	235	241	247	253	260	266	272	278	284	291	297	303	309	315	322	328	334
236	242	249	255	261	268	274	280	287	293	299	306	312	319	325	331	338	344
243	249	256	262	269	276	282	289	295	302	308	315	322	328	335	341	348	354
250	257	263	270	277	284	291	297	304	311	318	324	331	338	345	351	358	365
257	264	271	278	285	292	299	306	313	320	327	334	341	348	355	362	369	376
265	272	279	286	293	301	308	315	322	329	338	343	351	358	365	372	379	386
272	279	287	294	302	309	316	324	331	338	346	353	361	368	375	383	390	397
280	288	295	302	310	318	325	333	340	348	355	363	371	378	386	393	401	408
287	295	303	311	319	326	334	342	350	358	365	373	381	389	396	404	412	420
295	303	311	319	327	335	343	351	359	367	375	383	391	399	407	415	423	431
304	312	320	328	336	344	353	361	369	377	385	394	402	410	418	426	435	443

Weight Watchers will also measure your BMI for you, but you need to go to their centers to do that. This service is part of Weight Watchers and the American Cancer Society's Great American Weigh In. The two groups are working together to help people learn about the links between BMI and health risks, and to teach them how to lower BMI.

There are some limits to the BMI scale. It may overestimate body fat in athletes and others who have a muscular build. It may underestimate body fat in older people and others who have lost muscle mass.

Calculate Your Waist Circumference and Waist-Hip Ratio

To determine your waist circumference, place a tape measure snugly around your waist at the smallest point between your lower rib margin and the beginning of your hips. For women, a circumference greater than 35 inches is a sign of risk for the metabolic syndrome. For men, the figure is 40 inches.

Now measure your hips at the widest point around your buttocks. Divide your waist measurement by your hip measurement to find your waist-hip ratio. For example, if your waist is 28 and hips 40, your ratio is 0.70. If your ratio is greater than 0.80 for women or 0.95 for men, you have too much fat around the middle. The target ratio is 0.76. This calculation, too, can be found online. At the same NIH Web site given earlier, you click in your waist and hip measurements and are given your ratio with a message that you are or are not at risk. A high waist-hip ratio is known to be a marker for insulin resistance, which stimulates the production of estrogen.

Body fat distribution, in addition to overall obesity, also seems to matter. Women with abdominal obesity, based on their waist-hip ratio typical of an insulin-resistant state (android obesity), appear to be at higher risk than women whose body fat is more evenly distributed over their body (gynoid obesity). Upper-body and visceral fat are typical of higher levels of insulin.

Measuring Visceral Fat Stores (VAT Fat)

Sometimes a person may not be overweight, but suspicious blood tests may lead us to do a CT scan to detect hidden fat in the body. Visceral adipose tissue (VAT) is the fat that accumulates around the internal organs in your middle. It is different from fat that accumulates under the skin. We can see this fat—such as a large layer of fat surrounding the liver—with a CT scan of special X-rays.

Blood Tests

Blood tests offer us many gauges of insulin resistance. Blood tests include fasting blood sugar, a two-hour glucose tolerance test, cholesterol (HDL and LDL), triglycerides, C-peptide, a marker associated with high insulin levels, and C-reactive protein (CR-P), a marker of the inflammatory state typical of insulin resistance.

In some cases, we test for insulin growth factors (IGF-1) and other molecules, such as binding proteins (IGF-BP-1, 2, 3) and cytokines (such as IL-I), proteins that regulate the inflammatory state. Some blood tests help us determine levels of the B vitamins, liver function, electrolytes, and protein metabolism.

Glucose Tolerance Test

The glucose tolerance test can be done a variety of ways but the oral glucose tolerance test is the most commonly used. After an overnight fast, you drink a solution containing a known amount of glucose. Blood is obtained before you drink the glucose solution, and blood is drawn again every thirty to sixty minutes after the glucose is consumed, for up to three hours. This measures insulin levels. Readings from 110 to 126 indicate impaired glucose tolerance—the inability to clear glucose because of impaired response to insulin. A reading above 126 indicates diabetes.

C-Reactive Protein (C-RP)

C-reactive protein (C-RP) is not normally present in the blood but appears in increasing levels when any inflammatory process occurs, particularly during acute infection or malignancy, when levels of C-RP quickly shoot from less than 10 mg/L (milligrams per liter) to 1,000 mg/L or more. Newer tests using a high-sensitivity C-RP, or cardio C-RP, have in many cases supplanted the older test. This measurement is a powerful predictor of risk of heart disease, perhaps even more so than cholesterol, reflecting the growing recognition of the role of inflammation on this condition. This high-sensitivity C-RP will also show the increased inflammation of insulin resistance and the metabolic syndrome. For these reasons we routinely take at least two measurements to confirm the presence of an elevated C-RP level in all cancer patients. This test is likely to play a growing role as a predictor of cancer. In the low range it is less than 1, moderate range 1 to 3, and high-risk range is greater than 3 mg/L. Physicians frequently measure C-RP but are unaware of ways to reduce the levels. Diet and increased weight have been linked to high levels of inflammatory patterns like C-RP.

People often have high levels of C-RP because they don't get enough magnesium in their diet. Between 50 and 75 percent of the population does not get enough magnesium, according to recent studies. Magnesium can be taken as a supplement, often combined with calcium. C-RP levels can also be lowered when the metabolic state is treated with nutrition and exercise this way:

✳ Mediterranean and low-glycemic diet

✳ Adequate magnesium (whole grains, nuts, green leafy
   vegetables)

✳ Increased omega-3 (cold-water fish, flax, canola, nuts) and
   lower omega-6 (corn oil) fatty acids

✳ Low intake of trans-fatty acid

✳ Antioxidant vitamins (A, E, folate, B_6, B_{12}, and C)

✳ Coenzyme Q_{10} with mixed tocopherols

✳ Statins (cholesterol-lowering medications such as Lipitor)

✳ Aerobic fitness (short bursts of exercise may increase C-RP)

Blood Lipid Profile

A lipoprotein profile determines how much cholesterol is in your
blood. This tells us about total cholesterol: low-density lipoproteins (LDL, or bad cholesterol that builds up blockages); and high-
density lipoproteins (HDL, good cholesterol that helps prevent this
buildup; and triglycerides, another form of fat in your blood.

Cholesterol

Cholesterol is a fatty substance found in the blood and all cells
of the body. It is a critically important component in helping to
form cell membranes, steroid hormones, and other essential tissues. Over time, however, too much in the blood creates deposits of
fat on the walls of your arteries.

Thinking in terms of construction, cholesterol provides the
structural support of the "building." In your body, it provides the
structure to build cells that are needed to make hormones and
other body chemicals. When excess is made it clogs up the arteries.

There are two primary sources of cholesterol. The larger source
is produced in your body by your liver and is influenced by heredity as well as diet. A smaller component of cholesterol is derived
directly from the foods we eat. With rare exceptions (such as palm

oil), the majority of the food sources that increase cholesterol are from animal products. In both cases, it can be lowered by changes in diet and lifestyle and if necessary with medication, such as the statin drugs.

According to research done by the Mayo Clinic, about half of all Americans have a higher than desirable level of cholesterol. Nearly 105 million Americans age twenty and over have total blood cholesterol values of 200 mg/dL (milligrams per deciliter) or higher. This is about half the population. Only about 27 percent of the public knows what their cholesterol rate is or should be. Your LDL should be under 100. You should begin testing for cholesterol at the age of ten and then check it every five years. Starting at age forty, it should be checked every year.

Several physical and lifestyle factors contribute to high total cholesterol:

* Family history
* Diet high in saturated fats and cholesterol
* Weight (being overweight tends to increase cholesterol)
* Physical activity (regular exercise lowers the bad cholesterol and raises the good)

Low-density lipoprotein (LDL) is the primary carrier of cholesterol. Since too much LDL in the blood can lead to cholesterol buildup and block arteries, LDL is known as the "bad" cholesterol. High levels present an increased risk of heart disease. The amount of LDL in the blood is controlled in two important places: the liver, which produces cholesterol, using it to make digestive (bile) acids and remove cholesterol from the blood; and the intestine, which absorbs cholesterol that comes from food and from bile.

High-density lipoprotein (HDL) carries a third to a quarter of the cholesterol in the blood. Some experts believe that HDL cholesterol actually works to slow the buildup of cholesterol, since it carries cholesterol away from the arteries to the liver to be expelled by the body. For this reason, HDL cholesterol is known as the "good" cholesterol. High levels of HDL seem to protect against heart attack and other cardiovascular complications.

Think of LDL as the garbage and the HDL as the waste-management system. It cleans up the trash created by LDL. In women, estrogen loss at menopause causes HDL levels to drop.

A healthy person's cholesterol numbers should be something like this:

* Total cholesterol: below 200 mg/dL
* LDL: below 130
* HDL: above 40
* Triglycerides: below 200

Diet, weight, age, gender, and heredity can affect your cholesterol level. But physical activity can lower LDL and raise HDL.

Check www.2cholesterolsources.com for more information about cholesterol.

Triglycerides

Triglycerides are the principal fats—lipids—a mixture of fatty acids and glycerol circulating in your blood. Like cholesterol, triglycerides are necessary for life and provide much of the fuel needed for body cells to function. Triglycerides are derived from the food you eat: mainly sweets, red meat, dairy, and the liver itself, especially during times when dietary fats are not available. Calories ingested in a meal and not used immediately by tissues are converted to triglycerides and transported to fat cells to be stored. Hormones regulate the release of triglycerides from fat tissue so they meet the body's needs for energy between meals.

HDL, the good cholesterol, and triglycerides are related. It seems common for people with high triglycerides to have low HDLs.

High levels of sugar in the blood because of diabetes or insulin resistance cause triglyceride levels to rise. This can also be caused by prolonged stress, lack of exercise, long-term fasting, drinking too much alcohol, using hormones or steroids, and from a number of diseases. And when you have cancer, your triglyceride levels must be checked approximately every two months to see if chemotherapy is affecting them. Elevated triglycerides may be a consequence of disease such as untreated diabetes and cancer.

For eight to ten hours before the tests, you can have only water. In addition, no alcohol can be consumed for twenty-four hours before the test. Significant alterations in the fatty-acid pattern persist in the blood 24 hours after the consumption of alcohol. Anything you eat or drink other than water during that time can elevate the triglycerides, as they change dramatically in response to meals, increasing as much as five to ten times higher than fasting levels just a few hours after eating. However, even fasting levels may vary considerably from day to day.

Fat cells in the abdomen release fat into the blood more easily than fat cells found elsewhere. Release of fat begins three to four hours after the last meal, compared to many more hours for other fat cells. This easy release shows up as higher triglyceride and free-fatty-acid levels. Free fatty acids themselves can cause insulin resistance. We'll talk more about this in the next chapter.

The National Cholesterol Education Program, a division of the National Institutes of Health, has released the following recommendations of who should be treated for elevated triglyceride levels. Here is their policy on fasting blood triglyceride levels for adults.

If your triglyceride level is . . .	It is . . .
Less than 150 mg/dL	Normal
150–199	Borderline high

200–499	High
Over 500	Very high

Think of triglyceride levels in your blood as you would think of fat in milk. Normal is like 1 percent milk. Borderline compares to 2 percent milk. High is like whole milk, and very high compares to half-and-half.

It is fairly easy to reduce triglyceride levels by making lifestyle changes:

* Cut down on calories from all sources.
* Reduce saturated fats and cholesterol.
* Reduce alcohol intake.
* Be physically active for at least thirty minutes on most days.
* Eat fish high in omega-3 fatty acids.

Cortisol Function Test

Cortisol is a steroid hormone produced by the adrenal glands. It helps maintain blood pressure and cardiovascular function, reduces the immune system's inflammatory response, balances the effects of insulin in breaking down sugar for energy, and regulates metabolism of proteins, carbohydrates, and fats. One of cortisol's most important jobs is to help the body respond to stress. For this reason, women in their last three months of pregnancy and highly trained athletes normally have high levels of the hormone. People suffering from depression, alcoholism, malnutrition, panic disorder, and cancer also have increased cortisol levels.

Adrenocortical function is a fancy name for finding out how the adrenal glands are working to produce cortisol. We can check cortisol levels by taking saliva samples morning and night to find out how stressed—or not—you are by your cancer diagnosis. This testing can help us assess the impact of stress on response to the disease.

Did you know two pounds of saliva flows from your mouth each day? That usually shocks people. Saliva lubricates your throat and helps you swallow. It also contains enzymes that break down carbohydrates and antibacterial agents that help fight infection. And it's fast becoming the diagnostic specimen of choice for measuring levels of cortisol circulating in the body.

Only the free bioactive portion of a steroid hormone is filtered through the saliva ducts. This makes salivary cortisol a better indicator of adrenal activity than total blood levels. Unlike a blood draw, saliva collection is stress free, so the procedure itself does not affect the test results as a blood drawing might. In addition, multiple daily samples can be obtained, allowing us to determine any change in the daily secretion pattern. This helps us identify the need for additional intervention and also to time treatments such as chemotherapy.

Finding the Biorhythm of Chronic Stress

Many people with advanced cancer may be remarkably well adjusted to their disease, despite the difficulties of treatment and their guarded future. It is when we look at the physiologic measures of stress in this disease that the adverse effect on prognosis becomes evident. Everyone needs to be carefully assessed by their doctors for their psychological response to their cancer. It is no longer an issue of quality of life but important in treatment outcomes.

For example, cortisol rhythm may have a great deal to do with breast cancer outcome. According to a recent study in the *Journal of the National Cancer Institute,* it's not how much total cortisol the body secretes, but rather whether secretion follows a healthy up-and-down daily rhythm that appears closely tied to breast cancer survival. This blunted cortisol rhythm suggests an out-of-kilter stress response associated with poorer sleep patterns, loss of marital and social support, and increased sensitivity to stressors, all of which may affect survival rates.

Healthy people will have a rhythmic pattern of cortisol that rises early in the day to make you wake up and get moving. Those with an abnormal, flattened cortisol rhythm, typical for chronic stress, were found in a Stanford University study of more than one hundred women with metabolic syndrome to have a shortened survival from cancer. A study of two hundred colon cancer patients had similar results. (There is more about this in chapter 14 about sleep disruption in cancer treatment.)

An alteration in the hypothalamic-pituitary-adrenal axis leads to an abnormal cortisol rhythm in the adrenal gland and increased visceral fat storage. This has important implications for the relationship between severe stress and cancer outcomes, as well as adverse response to treatment.

Cortisol also suppresses your immune response by reducing natural killer-cell activity. Previous studies suggest that imbalances could cause tumors to grow faster. Interestingly, however, a disrupted cortisol rhythm still remained a "robust prognostic indicator of survival time" even after these related variables were considered.

By assessing the rhythm of cortisol in the saliva, we can better identify the need for additional interventions and we can time treatments such as chemotherapy more effectively. Excessively elevated morning salivary cortisol levels are often a sign of stress. In addition, normal blood cortisol measurements at 8 A.M. are high and at 4 P.M. are low. When these differences diminish, this altered diurnal pattern reflects significant stress.

Everyone needs to be carefully assessed by their doctors for their psychological response to their cancer. It is no longer an issue of quality of life but important in treatment outcomes.

The Psychological and Stress Profile

Having cancer is stressful and this stress sets in motion biological changes that can interfere with your cancer treatment and risk of recurrence. However, people vary in how they express their concern about having cancer. We spend time with each patient to see just how stressed they are. An initial baseline assessment helps us determine stress and psychological impact of the illness and each patient's coping style. How do they cope? Is the stress in proportion to the level of the illness? There are several tests that help us find out.

All cancer patients should be screened for stress. This includes depression, anxiety, fear, hopelessness, and helplessness. These are all prognostic markers to the doctor. The role of depression and anxiety on outcomes after heart attack and coronary bypass surgery is well accepted by cardiologists. Oncologists, on the other hand, are very adept at recognizing physical complaints among their patients but generally less skilled at identifying depression or anxiety. In one study of 204 cancer outpatients, oncologists were aware of the physical complaints in 80 percent of their patients, but failed to recognize clinical anxiety in 83 percent and clinical depression in 94 percent of affected patients. This reflects both inadequate training and the lesser importance placed on psychosocial stress by oncologists as a target for attention.

What Is Your Mental Adjustment to Cancer (MAC)?

Two well-known psycho-oncologists, Steven Greer and Maggie Watson, from the Royal Marsden Hospital in England, were interested in how patients' responses to cancer influenced their well-being and outcome with cancer. They sought a simple but reliable measure of patient response that was valid and could be self-administered by the patients themselves, making it a valuable clinical tool rather than a formal testing vehicle. From this MAC questionnaire they were able to define clusters of response that reflected five distinct coping styles in dealing with cancer. These included:

* Fighting spirit, the most common response, typified by a positive attitude, seeing life and their illness as a challenge
* Helpless, seeing life as hopeless and themselves as helpless to control events
* Fatalistic, accepting their condition and leaving it to their doctors; feeling nothing they do will make a difference
* Anxious preoccupation, fearing cancer's return or progression
* Avoidance or denial, feeling they don't really have cancer or denying its significance

Subsequent studies in breast cancer patients suggested that the helpless and hopeless response to cancer was particularly associated with an adverse outcome independent of the stage or grade of the cancer.

These scales are based on simple questionnaires that doctors can use in talking with patients. The scores help the doctor understand the patient's coping style. Is this person a fighter or helpless? Does he or she show anxious preoccupation, fatalism, or denial? Most people score between fighting spirit and preoccupation, followed by hopelessness.

Here are some statements doctors look for with the MAC. See if you identify with any of them:

* I have been doing things to improve my health.
* I feel I cannot do anything to cheer up.

* ❋ I believe I will get better.
* ❋ Nothing I do will help.
* ❋ I have plans for the future.
* ❋ I'm leaving it up to my doctor.
* ❋ I'm leaving it up to God.
* ❋ I feel like giving up.
* ❋ I see this as a challenge.
* ❋ I don't really believe I have cancer.

From a series of forty questions that the patients answer, the predominant coping response can be determined. It is particularly important to help patients who feel hopeless or out of control. Very often, individual counseling and group support can help. Doctors, too, can help by providing realistic but hopeful information. Without a crucial sense of hope, compliance with treatment, the quality of daily life, and, potentially, outcomes diminish.

ONCE THE metabolic profile is completed, we can plan the best possible treatment for each individual. We will be able to gauge the effects of the patient's body chemistry on the drugs, radiation, and surgery. We will know who will or will not respond to other medications used to reduce side effects of cancer treatment. We will be able to prescribe individual plans for diet, exercise, and stress reduction that will enhance cancer treatment and thus improve the outlook.

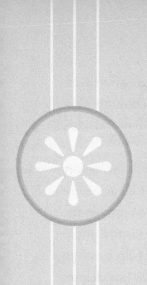

CHAPTER 3

How
Integrative
Cancer Therapy
Works

INTEGRATIVE CANCER THERAPY MESHES the best of conventional medical care with the best and most appropriate complementary therapy. With integrative therapy, doctors can help your body and mind to function together and at their best during cancer treatment. For instance, you can learn more about how the food you eat affects not only your general health, but the way you will respond to treatment. By learning ways to reduce the stress of cancer care, you make it more effective. This is total care, and it gives you all the tools necessary to overcome cancer and return to full health. Integrative therapy enables you to assist in your treatment.

In my practice, once we have given a cancer patient a complete workup, including a metabolic profile, we decide what he or she needs to treat the cancer. We make a treatment plan to cure the cancer if it is an early-stage tumor or to stop the progression of advanced cancer and its side effects. Once the surgery, chemotherapy, or radiation treatment is worked out, we plan nutrition, exercise, and stress-reduction treatment protocols.

Integrative treatment goals include reducing symptoms before treatment begins by using behavioral intervention with guided imagery, hypnosis (if needed), and other stress-reduction techniques. This way, the medical treatment itself will be more effective. If patients need surgery, there are special programs to help them go through it with as little anxiety and stress as possible (see chapter 11). A nutritional assessment should be made and patients should get started on individualized exercise training so they will be ready to continue it on a regular basis after surgery and during their chemotherapy or radiation treatment. In my practice we invite all of our patients to join a family support group.

These interventions continue during treatment. Nutrition includes monthly and biweekly follow-up visits. The same goes for symptom-reduction training and exercise. If patients have chemotherapy every two or three weeks, then we also confer with them about their nutrition, exercise, and stress-reduction programs. We want to know if they are sticking with the program or if they are having problems because of cancer treatment side effects.

If you have advanced cancer, you may require additional complementary therapies. For example, you may have more extreme side effects from higher-dose chemotherapy or radiation treatment and you may need liquid meals like ProSure and other supplements that will provide the vitamins and nutrients you need. The state of mind of the advanced cancer patient even before treatment begins is of special concern. Anxiety and depression need to be eased with mind-body techniques such as guided imagery, massage, or acupuncture, so that your cancer treatment will be more effective. You may also need additional conventional drugs for pain, inflammation, and the metabolic syndrome. Transfusions and antibiotics may also be part of therapy.

Once cancer treatment is completed, a medical management plan should be made. At this point, your cancer should be restaged for follow-up monitoring and interventions. For example, if the cancer was at stage 2 at the start of your treatment, you need to know if that has changed. A restaging workup should be done, including physical measurements, scans (CT), tumor marker levels, and lab tests to determine whether the inflammatory state or insulin resistance has changed and to look for lingering signs of cancer. And you should not leave your doctor's care without instructions in prevention, nutrition, and exercise to follow for the rest of your life. In our practice, we never let any patient fall off the cliff (see chapter 15).

Our cancer patients all have access to a biweekly and monthly family nutrition group program with a doctor, nutritionist, and nurse practitioner. Such visits help with nutritional reinforcement. So you see, in addition to basic medical treatment for cancer, you need specific plans to assure there are no long-term side effects from cancer or its treatment. Some of these conditions are explained below.

Limiting Weight Gain

Contrary to most people's understanding, many cancer patients gain rather than lose weight, particularly with chemotherapy for early-stage cancers such as breast. This is a common problem and a major concern because of the risk of disease progression, new cancers, and the development of other conditions, such as heart disease. There is evidence that the postchemotherapy fatigue syndrome may be linked to weight gain after treatment. All of these conditions may result in the rise in insulin levels, as well as estrogen and other mediators linked with weight gain.

In the Women's Healthy Eating and Living Study, researchers from Kaiser Permanente in California studied "low energy reporting," a measure of fatigue in breast cancer survivors. Women who had a BMI greater than 30 (indicating obesity) had twice the risk of low energy. Those women who gained weight during treatment had one and a half times the risk of fatigue by this index compared to those with stable weight following treatment. The two seem to be connected.

Before chemotherapy begins, as well as during and after, careful attention should be paid to weight gain. Changes in BMI, waist circumference, and waist-hip ratio must be monitored. Changes in fasting glucose, insulin, and lipids, particularly triglycerides and HDL cholesterol, should be followed. These provide relatively accurate indicators of the level of development of the insulin-resistant state and guide our nutritional interventions. Nutrition and exercise prescriptions should be provided even for patients who don't show signs of insulin resistance. This will limit its development and make sure those patients know how to maintain a self-care program.

At fifty, John was diagnosed with an acute and often fatal leukemia. He had high-dose chemotherapy and was free of leukemia for a year. When it recurred he had a bone-marrow transplant and was healthy for more than two years. Then at age fifty-four John had a stroke. Before his original diagnosis, John was active in sports and maintained a good diet and weight. His neurologist was unable to explain the stroke because there was no hypertension and arterial studies showed no sign of blood clotting. I noted, however, that John had extremely high levels of triglycerides and mildly elevated glucose levels. He had also gained twenty pounds in those three years and now did little exercise. While his total cholesterol count was normal at 190, his HDL had dropped to 38 from a high of 55. We discovered signs of insulin resistance not previously noted. Lab studies confirmed evidence of the metabolic syndrome with elevated insulin levels.

As is sometimes seen, aggressive chemotherapy can lead to the metabolic syndrome, which is clearly linked to a higher risk of stroke and heart disease. After six months on a program of weight reduction, exercise, and stress reduction, John's cholesterol, triglycerides, and insulin levels were back to normal.

An important *additional* reason for the diet and exercise program is to avoid the risk of cardiovascular disease due to chemotherapy-induced insulin resistance after curing cancer. Chemotherapy may induce the metabolic syndrome and affect overall prognosis, not just cancer. Keeping the metabolic syndrome under control is a win-win program.

Every researcher who has recognized the effect of cancer treatment on a patient's future believes cancer survivors must be advised of this risk of weight gain. You need to participate in a more active lifestyle and healthy diet to mitigate this potentially dangerous effect along with a lifelong follow-up to identify the development of the metabolic syndrome early.

Clinical trials of nutrition counseling and exercise are also in progress to find out how diet and exercise affect metabolism. When you gain weight with chemotherapy, more fat is added to the body while lean muscle mass declines at the same time. Multidrug chemotherapy is especially implicated in weight gains of five to fifteen pounds in postmenopausal women. Not only does this add fat and reduce muscle, it has an adverse emotional and social affect, too, as well as affecting survival.

When Patricia was diagnosed with breast cancer that had metastasized to her bones, she was nearing menopause and was thirty pounds over her ideal weight. She also had a stressful executive job as well as family problems. She began a chemotherapy regimen with Taxol and achieved a remission of her cancer over six months, but she also gained five more pounds. We then gave her a hormonal agent, Arimidex, to decrease production of estrogen in her body. Nevertheless, blood tests showed the level of cancer cells in her body had slowly begun to rise and she was uncertain what to do next when she came to see me.

A metabolic profile showed elevated insulin levels. Her BMI was 30. She had a high waist-hip ratio, as well as high levels of triglycerides and cholesterol. We put Patricia on a weight-reduction diet and began a stress-reduction program with meditation, guided imagery, and massage. Patricia's weight went down and her energy went up. Her insulin level normalized and remained stable. She continued with both weight training and aerobic exercise and remained stable on Arimidex. There is no evidence of progression of the disease through blood tests or on bone scans.

By normalizing her insulin, Patricia has had improvement in her response to treatment with Arimidex. This case is just a glimpse of the potential that lifestyle intervention has and its impact on breast cancer progression. We can't promise cure, but there is clear evidence that it is working.

Don't consider a few extra pounds unimportant. Work out a program with your doctor. Decide on your ideal weight (see the BMI chart) and stick to it with sensible diet and exercise—and stress reduction. Even a modest reduction in weight can reap significant benefits in terms of improving your metabolic status.

Limiting Weight Loss (Cancer Cachexia)

Cancer cachexia is a form of anorexia caused by cancer. It is among the most debilitating and life-threatening aspects of cancer. Like anorexia, cancer cachexia causes fat and muscle tissue to waste away, causing psychological distress and lowering the quality of life. It arises from a complex interaction between the cancer and the body that results in a chemical alteration of the metabolism. Cachexia is not caused by diet or anything else that the patient does. It is a condition where protein is broken down too fast by the body and thus the body suffers from advanced protein malnutrition. Any cancer patient with an involuntary weight loss of more than 5 percent of body weight within a six-month period is suspected to have this syndrome. I suspect cachexia in anyone losing weight at a higher rate than normal. They have hypermetabolism with abnormal insulin response and weight loss accompanied by insulin resistance. By testing the amount of albumin, the major circulating protein, in the blood of someone with a significant weight loss, we can recognize this condition.

Up to half of all advanced cancer patients may suffer from this syndrome at some time. Those with breast cancer or blood cancers get this less often but many patients with solid tumors may be at risk. About 80 percent of patients with upper-gastrointestinal cancers and 60 percent of those with lung cancer have already lost a substantial amount of weight by the time they are diagnosed.

Cachexia is also more common in children and the elderly and becomes more pronounced as the cancer progresses. The depression accompanying cancer may impair appetite and cause further weight loss. Despite normal intake of high-calorie foods, weight loss may continue because of the body's relentless breakdown of tissue protein. A multidimensional program of medical and behavioral interventions is needed. Omega-3 fatty acid supplements can aid nutrition status. Antidepressant drugs can be used to quell anxiety and bring insulin response back to normal and help the patient get needed nourishment. Ultimately, the most important treatment for cancer cachexia is successful control of tumor growth with conventional medical therapy.

Decreasing Insulin Resistance

Women with high levels of insulin (such as diabetics or those who are overweight and insulin resistant) may not respond as well to the anticancer effects of hormone treatments like tamoxifen. We now know that elevated levels of insulin growth factors such as IGF-1 may interfere with chemotherapy, even with the new drug Herceptin, a monoclonal antibody active against HER-2/neu-positive breast cancers. Lab studies are showing us that if we block these growth factors with compounds such as antibodies that bind and then activate them, we can potentially restore tumor sensitivity to Herceptin.

The insulin-like growth factors enhance survival of breast cancer cells after exposure to chemotherapy, thereby blocking programmed cell death. This happens with drugs such as 5-fluorouracil, cisplatin, Adriamycin, cyclophosphamide, and even Herceptin. To further complicate matters, dexamethasone, a steroid often given to combat nausea from chemotherapy, increases insulin levels by raising glucose and enhancing insulin resistance. So there is an obvious need to combat these effects as part of cancer therapy.

In men, prostate cancer is the major hormone-driven cancer. It is a disease of aging so the longer the prostate is exposed to androgens—the male hormones—the greater the long-term risk of cancer. This situation is similar in many ways to breast cancer, particularly in postmenopausal women, in which the breast ducts become sites for cellular changes caused by the long-term exposure to estrogen. Additional evidence is also showing an association with visceral obesity and increased BMI and prostate cancer. Moreover, numerous studies have implicated overweight and obesity with increasing prostate cancer mortality.

A study of 41,000 men aged forty to seventy in Australia linked more aggressive cancer with abdominal fat. Aggressive cancer in overweight men in nine military hospitals was studied from 1987 to 2002 following prostate surgery. The BMI was a predictor of higher-grade tumor, associated with a higher risk of recurrence and rising PSA levels after surgery.

All men should try to control their weight, whether or not they have cancer. If you have cancer, maintain a good weight to prevent recurrence and make the treatment more effective.

It is imperative in treating patients with insulin resistance that we correct that condition with diet and exercise and, especially, stress reduction.

Avoiding Postchemotherapy Fatigue Syndrome

One of the most common residual problems for women with breast cancer is persistent fatigue often accompanied by muscle and joint pain that sometimes mimics fibromyalgia. This has been blamed on many things, including posttreatment depression and anxiety. It is often short-lived, but in some women it can persist for months or even years.

Recent studies suggest a low-grade inflammatory state and elevated circulating cytokines as possible causes of postchemotherapy fatigue syndrome. A study of forty breast cancer survivors at the University of California at Los Angeles compared twenty women with this chronic fatigue and twenty without. They sampled blood for a variety of inflammatory cytokines and immune cells. The women with persistent fatigue had an increase in these body chemicals, so it was concluded that this posttreatment fatigue is caused by activation of inflammation and immune function.

This fatigue may begin in the early months of chemotherapy and may last for months or years after the end of chemotherapy. In contrast to women with advanced cancer who remain on a variety of cancer treatments, breast cancer survivors with fatigue are generally not anemic. Anemia is a common cause of fatigue in patients with metastatic cancer. It may be accompanied by sleep disruption and moodiness. Often, depression and anxiety go with it and are sometimes blamed for the condition. Despite its prevalence, it has received little attention until recently.

In a telling article in the journal *Oncology*, Marion Gilbert, forty-five and a breast cancer survivor, described her incapacitating fatigue, which persisted for eighteen months after her treatment ended. She said none of her doctors or other health-care professionals mentioned this side effect. Many of my own patients say that if they know what to expect, they are in a much better position to deal with the effects rather than being blindsided by them. This is especially important since the postchemotherapy fatigue syndrome may respond to a formal exercise program, such as daily vigorous walking or low level-aerobics. You should increase, not decrease, your activity. There's more about how to fight fatigue in chapter 10.

Risks after Childhood Cancer

Because of the growing success of chemotherapy and radiation for childhood malignancies such as acute leukemia and testicular cancer, there are lots of long-term survivors reaching adulthood. We know now they are vulnerable to chronic illness such as cardiac disease and second cancers and three times more vulnerable to premature death than the general population. This is linked to intense chemotherapy and radiation.

These survivors are also at risk of obesity and the metabolic syndrome and this contributes to the above-mentioned risks. A group of childhood leukemia survivors who had had bone-marrow transplant were followed in a study by the University of Helsinki in Finland. More than half had insulin resistance, with 39 percent showing signs of the metabolic syndrome. Part of this effect is blamed on the radiation to the nervous system commonly used in the treatment of childhood acute leukemia, which results in a deficiency of growth hormone and secondary insulin resistance. In a similar study in England, both boys and girls surviving acute lymphoblastic leukemia, the most common form, had a 50 percent chance of being obese young adults. There are many long-term survivors reaching adulthood.

SO YOU can see why integrative therapy and a long-term therapy plan are needed. In the following chapters on nutrition, exercise, and stress reduction, you will learn the various ways this can be achieved. These interventions will not only make your cancer treatment more effective, they will improve your future health and well-being as a cancer survivor.

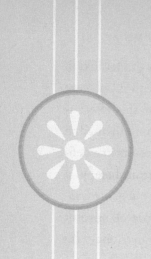

CHAPTER 4

How Targeted Nutrition Makes Cancer Treatment More Effective

NOW THAT YOU UNDERSTAND how my program works, I want you to take a serious look at nutrition. For most patients, cancer is a wake-up call to eat in a more healthful way. This is more serious than simply trying to lower your cholesterol or cut out the salt. You want to make sure you are doing everything you can to assure a long life.

Like most Americans, you are probably confused about diet and cancer. Studies proclaim the benefits of broccoli and other cruciferous vegetables to ward off breast cancer or cooked tomatoes to prevent prostate cancer. We were told to eat less fat and as a result we ate more carbohydrates. Then we heard that carbs were bad and fat was okay. Medical science has been focusing on individual foods, but it's becoming clear that overall nutrition pattern and its relationship to body weight and activity are what really matter.

A sound nutrition plan is necessary during and after treatment, not only to prevent the return of your cancer, but also to:

* Reduce the oxidative state, often caused by chemotherapy
* Reduce the inflammatory state
* Reduce the metabolic syndrome or prevent its development
* Treat side effects

The next few chapters will help you make a dietary plan. But first, let's look at how we got so confused about nutrition.

Learning from the Hunter-Gatherers: The Paleolithic Diet

In the preagricultural days of the hunter-gatherers, over ten thousand years ago, men and women ate what was growing naturally on trees, shrubs, and in the fields. This included nuts, tuberous vegetables, and edible fruits. Some anthropologists believe that the development of color vision in higher primates was designed to allow early man to identify ripe and highly edible fruits when they were most nutritious and appropriate for picking. Because they contained highly concentrated fructose, fruits were a valuable source of calories, when available.

Free-ranging wild game was lean and muscular, in contrast to the meat we eat today that is grown in stockyards and fed with processed grains and fattened with hormones. There were no mass-produced chickens grown in cubicles and fed with artificial foods and antibiotics to enhance growth. People ate only wild fowl and birds they were able to catch, often requiring a significant amount of physical exertion to obtain. Recent studies of the Paleolithic diet now suggest that a much higher proportion of the diet was composed of this animal protein, including fish where available. Today, it is only the rare hunter who brings home venison who gets this healthier meat. In contrast to today's porterhouse steak, this meat is rich in omega-3 fats (more typical of salmon), known to help prevent cancer and protect the heart.

The Paleolithic Diet

There are about eighty-four tribes of hunter-gatherers still in existence. Many are isolated in predominantly tropical areas of South America, Asia, southern Africa, and Australia. Few of these tribes have not been affected by encroaching civilization and the inevitable changes in their hunter-gatherer lifestyles. They are generally slim and muscular, stronger and faster than people living in industrialized Western countries, and have excellent eyesight and remarkably healthy teeth. Cancer, diabetes, heart disease, depression, and other maladies of the modern world are for the most part rare. It is not unusual for members of these tribes to live well into elderly years.

Many of these tribes still eat the way hunter-gatherers did for the last fifty thousand years. Despite encroaching civilization, they continue to maintain a lifestyle typical to one they were originally developed for. We have all evolved from this diet and our adaptation to this life is encoded within our genes.

The anthropologist James Neel suggested that early man had a predisposition to store excessive calories as fat when they were available. This he termed the "thrifty phenotype." When people ate lots of protein and limited carbohydrates, their bodies needed a way to maintain adequate blood sugar in the face of this low-carbohydrate diet. So when they did have a chance to eat carbohydrates, such as the berries of summer, the insulin level would rise, resulting in the conversion of sugar to triglyceride for fat storage. These fat stores can be called upon when food supplies are low. This was particularly important for women who were nursing or carrying babies and needed glucose for the growing fetus and for the newborn.

Whatever the case, our original premodern diets, typical of Paleolithic man and our prehuman ancestors, existed for hundreds of thousands of years and it is only in the last several hundred years—particularly with the advent of modern food processing in the last fifty years—that our diets have so drastically changed. This led to a dramatic alteration in our pattern of illness. Because we have been adapted over many millennia to this Paleolithic background, it is understandable that we have a limited genetic adaptation to our new lifestyle.

This early Paleolithic diet was rich in lean meat from game, occasionally supplemented by eggs, fruits, nuts, and vegetables and also accompanied by fish in those populations living near water. There were no grains, milk, beans, soy, or lentils and certainly no refined sugar. These diets were high in quality protein, very high in fiber, and rich in vitamins, minerals, iron, omega-3 fats, mono- and polyunsaturated fats, and abundant in nutrients and antioxidants. They were also low in salt and saturated fat.

Among those aboriginal hunter-gatherer societies that have survived into the twenty-first century, the rates of cancer, obesity, diabetes, and heart disease are remarkably low. When these tribes switch to more modern diets, the incidence of these illnesses rises with them. Thus, many nutritionists believe a Paleolithic diet and lifestyle might be an effective weapon against the adverse effects of modern affluence, reducing the risk of cancer, heart disease, and obesity. Obviously, we're not going to go hunting, fishing, and berry picking, but we can certainly eat foods that fit within this standard.

The Mediterranean Diet

The Mediterranean diet developed after the Paleolithic Age but well before modern industrial times. Agriculture was first limited to fruits and nuts that grew on trees and the harvesting of olives that is the characteristic of the Mediterranean basin. Domestication of animals soon followed. It has been well documented that people in the Mediterranean regions, despite a high level of smoking, live longer than those from other areas of Europe. And it is not simply genetic because studies show that non-Mediterranean populations receive the same benefits when consuming the typical diet of that region.

The benefits of the Mediterranean diet extend to populations living throughout the Mediterranean basin, from southern Spain, France, and Italy to Greece, Turkey, Crete, and extending along the northern African coast. Traditional Mediterranean diets, in contrast to northern European and American diets, include a significantly larger amount of plant foods, rich in protective nutrients and antioxidants. These are found in fruits, vegetables, nuts, wholegrain cereals, olive oil and olives, and moderate amounts of wine.

Even today the Mediterranean diet not only produces favorable cholesterol and lipid levels, but also protects against oxidative damage to cells, which is thought to be one of the mechanisms leading to chronic illness such as cancer. The preference for fresh fruit and vegetables means that more raw foods are eaten. Thus, there is a lower production of cooking-related oxidative compounds. When you eat more fruit and vegetables, you get more antioxidants and nutrients (such as flavonoids and polyphenols) as well as very high fiber.

Less Cancer in the Mediterranean

The incidence for cancer overall in Mediterranean countries is lower than that of northern Europe and the United States. They have lower rates of cancer of the colon, breast, uterus, and prostate. These forms of cancer have been linked to low consumption of fruits and vegetables and higher consumption of meat, unlike the typical Mediterranean diet. Mortality statistics from the World Health Organization, as well as other studies, clearly document the low incidence for most cancers and the longer survival overall of the people within the Mediterranean region, even with the high prevalence of smoking.

A recent study by Harvard and the Pfizer Company found that Spanish women live longer than any other Europeans and their diet rich in olive oil may be the reason. The Spanish use more olive oil than any other country in the world. The study pointed to the concentrations of resveratrol and flavones in olive oil along with Spain's good health-care system. On average, Spanish women live 83.7 years, three years longer than women in the United Kingdom and nearly four years longer than American women.

In the groundbreaking Lyon Diet Heart Study, which examined the effect of the traditional Mediterranean diet on heart disease, researchers found a remarkable change in relationship to cancer. They compared people on a traditional Mediterranean diet with others on an American Heart Association heart disease prevention diet. In those on the traditional Mediterranean diet, not only was there a reduction in heart disease and death, *there was a 61 percent reduction in cancer death*. This study reinforces the known connection between a Mediterranean diet and reduced risk for many of these cancers.

The Western Diet and Cancer

When people migrate from the Mediterranean region to the United States or Australia, these patterns change, disproving the idea that cancer may be due to inherited differences among people in these populations. Within one generation of arriving at the new locations, more of these migrants die from these cancers. If we consider this, we can safely estimate that up to 25 percent of the cases of colorectal cancer, 15 percent of breast cancer, and 10 percent of prostate, pancreas, and endometrial cancer may be prevented if people in Western countries shifted to the traditional Mediterranean diet.

While cancer rates are still low in the Mediterranean area, the disease has been increasing. From the 1960s through the 1990s, breast, colon, and prostate cancer is on the rise along with rising urbanization and westernization of lifestyle. There's been a slow decline in the consumption of whole-grain cereals, although they continue to eat relatively high amounts of fruits and vegetables. However, even though olive oil remains a staple of the diet, there has been a marked increase in the consumption of animal fats, particularly meat.

A National Health and Nutrition Examination Survey looked at dietary patterns of healthy adults in the United States and their effects on insulin resistance and cardiovascular risk factors. People who had a Western pattern characterized by lots of processed meats, eggs, red meats, and high-fat dairy were compared with those with a Mediterranean-type American healthy pattern characterized by green leafy vegetables, tomatoes, cruciferous vegetables, and peas. Those who had the Western diet had high levels of C-peptide, a measure of chronic insulin production and higher blood sugar in the long term. This typical Western diet was clearly linked to a high risk of insulin resistance. The American healthy diet pattern reflects the increasing interest among the American population, particularly the younger, better educated, and more affluent who are eating more vegetables and fruit foods rich in fiber and less refined carbohydrates. In other words, more like the original Mediterranean diet.

However, there's still a long way to go. Most people still do not eat enough fruit and vegetables every day to get all the nutrients and fiber they need. In a thirteen-year American Institute for Cancer Research study led by the Mayo Clinic College of Medicine, the hardest thing for the survey participants to do was comply with the fruit and vegetable criteria. Only 11 percent of the thirty thousand postmenopausal women surveyed had five or more servings a day.

Nutrition's Future Role in Worldwide Cancer Prevention and Treatment

The World Cancer Research Fund International is working on a remarkable new study. In November 2003 they announced that an upcoming global report on nutrition, physical activity, and cancer prevention will employ an innovative method to review the data.

* Population studies will compare the preexisting diets and cancer rates of entire countries or regions.
* Migration studies will compare how cancer rates change when individuals eating a traditional regional diet move to a new country or region and adopt the local diet.
* Diets of a group of cancer patients in the years before diagnosis will be compared to the diets eaten in the same time

period by a group of statistically similar individuals who are
still cancer free.

✳   The existing diets and cancer rates of large groups of individuals will be tracked over several years.

When this study is completed in 2006 we will have new ways to set
nutritional goals for the world.

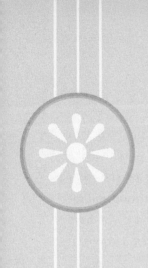

CHAPTER 5

Eating to Reduce the Metabolic Syndrome and Enhance Cancer Treatment

MANY OF MY PATIENTS, especially the women, have some knowledge of nutrition, or they show an interest in it. But, while people seem more interested in nutrition these days, there's still plenty of confusion. The popularity of low-carb diets is partly to blame. Patients tell me they don't want to eat fruit because of the sugar content, or they won't eat oatmeal because it's a carbohydrate. But the most interesting thing is that all of them agree that doctors often don't seem to know as much as they do about nutrition. One cancer specialist told a patient who was overweight and insulin resistant not to worry about her diet. "Don't do anything," he told her. She felt very let down by this, and rightly so.

Creating a Dietary Plan

Before treatment begins, you and your doctor should sit down with a nutritionist and discuss your dietary history so that you can make a feasible dietary plan. Your doctor needs to know how and what you eat, where you shop, whether or not you read nutrition and ingredient labels, what kind of restaurants you like, and if you have ever been on any fad diets. Ask yourself some of these questions:

* Are you allergic to any foods?
* Are you on a special diet for any other condition such as diabetes?
* Do you have financial, family, or cultural limitations regarding food?
* Do you have a natural aversion to anything?

One of my patients could never stand to eat bananas. The smell, texture, everything about them made her feel ill. She said if she ate a banana she would feel sick all day. Obviously, bananas as a source of potassium and fiber were not an option for her. A middle-aged man had been treated for diverticulitis years earlier and refused my suggestion of adding some flaxseeds to his morning cereal as a way to get omega-3 fatty acids. He was convinced the seeds would get stuck in his large intestine and cause problems. An attorney in my care refused to eat fish. He said all during his childhood he had been forced to eat fish on Fridays and hated it. Because he would not eat fish, we had to be sure he got his omega-3 fatty acids from another source, such as fish oil supplements. Economic factors may limit your food choices, too. People with modest incomes may use food stamps and thus be limited to where they can shop for food. Your dental history may come into play. Some people don't eat fresh fruits and vegetables because their teeth are not in good shape. They may want to eat only soft foods simply because it's more comfortable for them. Others may have teeth that are sensitive to cold or heat.

All of these factors must be considered in order to set nutritional goals.

Keep a Food Diary

The first step to setting nutritional goals is to keep a food diary for two weeks and write down everything you eat from the moment you wake up until bedtime, so that your dietary pattern can be assessed. Much as people often forget where their pennies go during the day and need to write it all down for budgeting purposes, few realize how much or even what they eat during the span of a day. By writing down everything you put in your mouth, you will quickly determine whether or not you are eating much more than you need and this very act will help reduce your level of consumption. You will also realize how often you eat when you are not hungry. This will help you to see the pattern of your eating and the kinds of food that may be lacking or excessive in your diet.

Once you have written it all down for two weeks and reviewed your eating history, it's time to create a dietary plan and nutritional supplement program. Notice I didn't say "diet." I don't put anybody on a diet. As soon as you hear diet, you think of deprivation and this causes stress. This is why fad diets never work in the long run. They make you think you can't eat the things you love. A dietary plan simply means you eat a variety of healthful and tasty foods in moderate amounts. With moderation and diversity, you are never deprived.

In my practice, we create feasible diet plans for weight maintenance and loss based on Mediterranean-style eating, including specific nutritional advice about chemotherapy, such as what to do when you are too nauseated to eat.

Biodiversity Is the Key to a Well-Balanced Diet

In your stock portfolio, diversity will keep you from losing your shirt and everything else. The key to health is in diet diversity. In fact, it's crucial. A fixed or rigid diet is not only boring, it adds to your stress level, thereby increasing cortisol secretion, and may elevate insulin levels regardless of what you eat. Variety lowers your risk of any one food having a negative effect on your health. It also keeps you interested and involved.

Nature has blessed the plant world and the foods we obtain from it with myriad valuable nutrients, vitamins, complex carbohydrates, and many important trace minerals. These vary from plant to plant, particularly between different plant families such as alliums (garlic and onions) and cruciferous plants (broccoli, cauliflower, Brussels sprouts). This rich mixture of nutrients is the crucial point in your dietary plan. Together they work to reduce cancer risk, in part through mechanisms that detoxify carcinogens. And the well-documented antioxidant effect of many nutrients, as well as the major role plant foods play in limiting obesity and the insulin-resistant state, are all part of this synergy.

The biodiversity dietary plan means the wider the variety, the greater the number of nature's medicines. This is so important to our future as cancer survivors. I recently noticed a food pyramid chart that groups foods by colors as a guide rather than by category such as vegetable or fat. The goal here is to mix up lots of colors, so the veggies synergize with one another.

Educate yourself about caloric density. One of the reasons for eating plenty of fresh fruits and vegetables is that they contain roughage and water and therefore make you feel full. You can eat lots more of them and therefore satisfy hunger with fewer calories. When you feel full, your brain receives signals to stop eating. You can easily fill up on soups and salads, which have lots of bulk and water, but are low in calories.

There's an important interaction between a diverse nutritious diet that limits weight gain and a lifestyle that includes regular, daily physical activity. This is the essence of the Mediterranean diet and lifestyle and shares many features of the Paleolithic diet. This is particularly important for the cancer survivor.

Don't Look for the Tree, Enjoy the Forest

For the last twenty years, science has been trying to identify those dietary components linked to specific cancers, such as fiber and colon cancer, or dietary fat levels and breast cancer. Subsequent studies suggested potential mechanisms, such as the alteration of estrogen metabolism by indole-3-carbinol, found in cruciferous vegetables like broccoli. Or they focus on the alteration in stool transit time or levels of short-chain fatty acids in the gut, resulting in less colon cancer from high-fiber diets. Despite these expectations, several large trials have failed to show an influence of fiber on the formation of colon polyps, the precancerous lesions that can lead to colon cancer if left in place. Similarly, several large studies of women followed carefully over years have failed to reveal a significant relationship between increased dietary fat intake and breast cancer.

And many of us don't get it. More than 75 percent of Americans still believe a specific kind of food is more important for losing weight than the sheer amount of food they eat. This feeds the erroneous belief that particular foods can prevent cancer. While it is true that the lycopene in cooked tomatoes helps prevent prostate cancer, and the phytonutrients in broccoli and other cruciferous vegetables help prevent breast cancer, these foods by themselves will not protect you if your overall pattern of nutrition is unbalanced.

Remember, it is the overall dietary pattern rather than any single constituent that is important. *Diet diversity is crucial*. A rigid diet followed compulsively may often increase stress, though its effect on higher cortisol levels and increased insulin may impair your ability to lose weight even while consuming fewer calories. This is why so many fixed diets are self-defeating. By an overly compulsive approach to dieting rather than attention to both diet pattern and overall lifestyle, including physical activity, weight loss and good health may be more difficult to attain. New diet books are constantly appearing because people are seeking a magic bullet. By eating less and moving more, and balancing fats, carbohydrates, proteins, and micronutrients, both weight loss and good health will follow.

Basic Nutritional Guidelines for Cancer Patients

A healthy diet is generally based on 25 percent protein, 30 percent fat (20 percent for prostate cancer patients) and 45 percent healthy (complex) carbohydrates. Here is a summary of these three food groups; the following chapters will give you specifics about each group along with lists of foods to choose and foods to avoid.

Carbohydrates

Fresh fruits and vegetables are the best kinds of carbohydrates to eat and should provide the bulk of your daily food intake. They provide vitamins, minerals, fiber, and antioxidants in a way that supplements simply cannot do. Use organic produce whenever possible. Get variety simply by using lots of different colors. Include leafy greens, red tomatoes and peppers, yellow squash, and so on. There is no end to the colors, flavors, and textures available. Eat legumes and beans as often as possible because they are high in vitamins, minerals, soluble fiber, and antioxidants, and low in calories and sodium.

Have *at least* five servings per day of vegetables and fruit but preferably more. Remember, a half cup to one cup of cooked or raw vegetables is one serving. So one large colorful salad a day could provide the five servings. (However, it's best to break that up into smaller meals.) Eat fruit in its natural state and avoid fruit juices with added sugars and preservatives.

Avoid concentrated carbohydrates such as sugar, honey, corn syrup, and refined starches like white bread and baked goods. Eat whole-grain breads and cereals, which are high in B vitamins, iron, and fiber. Limit pasta and potatoes. (The U.S. Potato Board is so concerned at the loss of potato sales because of the low-carb diet craze that they are developing a new potato with less carbohydrate.)

Protein

Most of your protein should come from poultry, fish, legumes, and low-fat dairy products. Limit lean red meat to twice a week. (Grilled red meat should be limited to once a week to avoid too much exposure to the carcinogens in the char.) Avoid the skin on poultry and buy free-range or organic when possible. Meat and poultry are high in B vitamins, iron, and other minerals. Eat cold-water fish with omega-3 fatty acids such as Pacific wild salmon once or twice a week but limit fish with high mercury content as well as those with high pesticide and pollution content, such as farm-raised salmon.

Eggs are high in protein, B vitamins, iron, and other minerals. The yolks are also high in cholesterol, so limit whole eggs to three times a week. Egg whites can be eaten more often.

Milk products are high in protein, calcium, phosphorus, niacin, riboflavin and vitamins A and D. Use skim milk, nonfat yogurt, and low-fat cheese.

Fats and Oils

You need fats to maintain healthy cells. Some of these fats are high in vitamins A or E, but all are high in calories. Use moderate to low saturated fats, no trans fats, and a balanced ratio of monounsaturated omega-3 fatty acids. We carefully teach our patients to understand the difference between good and bad fats (see chapter 7). Nuts are healthy fats more than they are fruits or a source of protein. Olives, too, are healthy fat.

Adjust your total fat intake to caloric needs. For example, if you are trying to lose weight then limit yourself to five teaspoons (one and a half tablespoons) of fat a day. That is less than twenty-eight grams. In general, serving sizes are one tablespoon of vegetable oil or seeds.

Fluids

Drink plenty of water, at least two quarts—eight eight-ounce glasses—a day. Keep in mind that alcohol does not count as a serving of fluid. It dehydrates you. In addition, using alcohol regularly can affect your treatment. Drink two to three cups of green tea as a way to get some of your fluids. Green tea has lots of healthful antioxidants, helps reduce insulin resistance, and it does not have as much caffeine as black tea. However, don't take green tea supplements. They are not regulated by the FDA and may contain fillers and contaminants.

Preventing Weight Gain or Loss

People who are on adjuvant curative chemotherapy account for the biggest population in my office. These are patients who have had surgery and are now involved in follow-up chemotherapy. From the get-go in my practice we begin nutritional intervention, which we monitor during and after treatment. If necessary, the nutritional program is planned with weight gain or loss in mind, as well as gastrointestinal side effects of treatment, and controlling the metabolic syndrome.

When you are being treated for cancer, it is even more important to understand how the food you eat as well as the amount you consume may affect your treatment. Most people are concerned about weight loss during treatment and fail to realize that in many cases it is the weight gain that often accompanies cancer and its treatment that may have adverse long-term effects. Nutrition is absolutely important during all phases of cancer treatment and follow-up. Your goal should be to avoid excess weight gain or loss while in treatment and after it ends.

Chemotherapy often reduces lean muscle mass while adding weight primarily from fat and water. This is called sarcopenic obesity. It occurs when there is a low BMI but an increased percentage of body fat. This means your weight for your height is normal or below normal and although you look thin, you have reduced lean body mass and increased body fat. This is not a healthy state because it increases your risk for cancer recurrence. It also reduces your tolerance to therapy. So it's important to avoid weight gain in the early stage of cancer. This is especially important in young people with cancer, a phenomenon that is unrecognized by most patients and doctors (see chapter 3).

Preventing Nausea, Food Aversions, and Food Cravings

Cancer treatment has a big effect on your ability to get proper nourishment. It can cause nausea and other digestive problems that limit your desire to eat. Food aversions and food cravings also develop during treatment. Some patients develop cravings for sugar, chocolate, and fats when on chemotherapy. This is not simply about wanting to eat something to make them feel good. Their body chemistry is mixed up and sending skewed signals. One of my patients undergoing chemotherapy for uterine cancer constantly craved chocolate ice cream, although she could hardly eat anything else. We suggested she give in to one scoop of this ice cream a day and try more appropriate foods at other times, such as sherbet or low-fat yogurt. Obviously, filling up on any of these cravings would be harmful, so we educate our patients and help them work through the craving by recommending other foods, urging them to drink lots of water, and using some of the guided imagery techniques. These cravings are quite common but they stop when chemotherapy stops. If you crave your favorite foods and then feel nauseated from them, then in later years you will always associate the food with that feeling. This is a learned conditioned response. Try new foods instead.

In addition, avoid spicy, oily, salty, and fried foods, all of which are more difficult to digest. Avoid foods with strong or pungent aromas because the smell alone will nauseate you.

Smaller, more frequent meals are important during therapy because when you are nauseated, it may be difficult to eat enough. In this case, you may need to take a liquid-diet supplement such as Boost, Ensure, or ProSure. The latter is one of the best because it has a good balance of omega-3 fatty acids. Another way to overcome the inability to eat is to try drinking shakes, juices, and smoothies to get the maximum nutrients. For example, if you have access to a juicing machine you can make juice from fresh carrots, peppers, parsley, and other vegetables for a synergistic variety of nutrients and antioxidants. The fresh aroma of the vegetables is less likely to bring on nausea, which often occurs when patients smell food cooking.

Ginger ale is often used as an antinausea drink.

Avoid lactose products if you have diarrhea, except for nonfat yogurt, which you should eat daily because it helps to balance the bowel flora. Increase fluids and fiber intake.

Acupuncture and acupressure also help some patients relieve gastrointestinal distress (see chapter 13).

Making Good Nutrition Part of Your Lifestyle

Shopping, preparing meals, and eating take up a considerable amount of time each day. And because it is time-consuming, people often cut corners when they are busy. As a result, even with the best intentions, we don't always get the best and most nutritious foods. There are ways to make shopping, preparing meals, and eating out more nutritious—and also a pleasurable part of our lifestyle.

Learning Portion Size

One of the most important things to learn in watching what and how you eat is how to determine portion size. Fill a measuring cup or spoon with your prescribed serving size and empty it out onto a clean plate or bowl. Do this once or twice and you will get a mental snapshot of what that serving size looks like.

A three-ounce piece of meat is about the size of a deck of cards. A portion of cooked vegetable is about the size of a baseball. A one-ounce serving of cheese looks like four dice. Eventually you learn how to eyeball it. The last thing we want you to do is become obsessed—and stressed out—with exact measurements. Here again, it would feel as if you were on a strict diet. This is not the case, but by doing some measuring in the beginning, you will get a much better sense of what portion sizes look like.

You may be surprised to know that the bowl of cereal you eat every morning contains twice or even three times the amount listed as a serving (and fat, calories, and sugar) than you think. For example, the nutrition label on the box may say a half cup of the cereal (without milk) has 210 calories and another forty calories with a half cup of skim milk added. However, most people just pour the cereal into a bowl without measuring and end up eating 520 calories of just the cereal. When they add milk (again, without measuring) they have a 600-calorie bowl of cereal. And even if it is made of healthful whole grains, it is still too much carbohydrate to eat at one sitting. Likewise, a tablespoon of olive oil confers several health benefits to a salad, not to mention about 125 calories. If you just pour it over a salad without measuring, you could triple the amount. If you use prepared salad dressings, even low-calorie ones, you will be surprised how many calories you will get if you don't teach yourself what a "portion" looks like.

You can also get a little calorie-counting handbook from your bookstore. These list all the foods you are likely to eat and tells you portion size, calories, and sometimes other content such as fat, carbohydrates, and protein.

The steady growth of American portion sizes directly contributes to the steady growth of people's weight. In the 1950s, a family-size bottle of Coke was twenty-six ounces. Today a single-serving bottle is twenty ounces. McDonald's original burger and fries with a twelve-ounce Coke provided 590 calories. A super-size extra value meal with a Quarter Pounder and cheese, super-size fries, and a super-size Coke delivered 1,550 calories (McDonald's no longer offers super-size menu items). A typical bagel used to weigh two to three ounces, but today is four to seven ounces.

More Americans than ever are eagerly polishing off whatever amount of food is in front of them. The new data confirm what experts feared. Americans have lost sight of the basic relationship between the portions we eat and the weight we carry and focus too exclusively on cutting out specific types of food, such as carbohydrates or fats.

According to the report, 69 percent of Americans now say that when dining at table-service restaurants, they finish their entrees most of the time, up 2 percent from 2000. The number of women who say this has doubled, from 9 to 18 percent. The American Institute for Cancer Research has been tracking the steady growth of portions in restaurants and fast-food outlets over the past twenty years.

Americans have even adopted this passive approach to portions at home, with 30 percent saying they generally based the amount of food they eat on the amount they are served. These are troubling findings in light of recent scientific studies that show that we can and do unconsciously consume more calories—as much as 56 percent more—when served larger portions.

Many people don't understand how the French eat so well (including high-fat sauces, cheeses, and other foods) without getting as fat as Americans. It has everything to do with portion control and attitude about food. The French appreciate the pleasure they get from their foods and rarely think about it in terms of health. They eat a more diverse diet of smaller portions—and they don't mind leaving some food on the plate. Americans, on the other hand, seem to be members of the clean-plate club.

Jacques Pépin, a well-known French-born American chef who understands nutrition as well as fine food, and many other people agree that we need to sit down to dinner with our families and enjoy the food we eat. Pépin, who inherited high cholesterol from his father, believes strongly that food can be delicious as well as nutritious. He has written many cookbooks about healthy—and tasty—meals. However, he says the pleasure of the meal is important and should be shared with others. American families spend less time eating together because of work and school schedules. They eat on the run more often and alone more often. Pépin suggests eating with others as often as possible. If you are feeling pleasure while eating, you are not experiencing stress. If you are rushing through your food and not really enjoying it, you are creating a stressful situation. Even eating less food could leave you with more fat, especially the abdominal fat caused by the stress hormone cortisol.

Eat Mini Meals

Six small, frequent meals may be better than three big meals for anyone, but when you are being treated with chemotherapy or radiation for cancer, it makes special sense. Large meals may be precluded by nausea, impaired appetite, or sore mouth. There is some evidence, though limited, that smaller but frequent mini-meals through the day may be metabolically advantageous and helpful in weight control, in contrast to the rigid three meals a day pattern typical for Americans.

The International Union of Nutrition Sciences studied older Greeks to evaluate the effect of eating patterns on obesity, diabetes, and cardiovascular risk. They looked at people who ate a greater number of meals or snacks each day; those who ate at least two cooked meals daily; and those having breakfast earlier rather than later in the morning. Here's what they found:

* Later dinner times in the evening were associated with higher blood sugar levels.
* A more varied diet was associated with a greater number of meals daily and lower risk of diabetes and heart disease (see biodiversity on page 64).
* People who had breakfast earlier rather than later in the morning were less obese.

This study suggests that the traditional Mediterranean diet with lots of vegetables, fruit, olive oil, cheese, fish, and wine, may contribute to lower levels of obesity and favor greater diet diversity.

In an additional study, overweight men who did not have diabetes ate either a single large meal or many smaller meals throughout the day. The total number of calories available was identical for each group and they were told to eat as much of the offered meal or meals as they wished. Despite an absence of hunger, those men given a single meal consumed 27 percent more calories than those provided with five small meals. In addition, those having the single large meal had higher peak insulin levels. Smaller, more frequent meals in this study resulted in fewer overall calories consumed and a lower insulin level. This reinforces the potential benefit for this meal pattern in limiting weight gain and thus insulin resistance.

While meal pattern and frequency may be important, the meal content is crucial. The typical American couch potato pattern of chips, cookies, and other fast-food snacks between large meals are clearly not part of this message. Rather, healthy small meals of fruit, yogurt, nuts, or cut vegetables such as carrots, and other easy-to-make midday snacks better reflect this healthy diet pattern. Eating more frequently keeps hunger at bay and puts less stress on the digestive system. When you eat small, calorie-dense meals, choose vegetables and fruits and drink lots of water.

Don't Skip Breakfast

Breakfast is important because it jump-starts your metabolism for the day and helps keep weight down. Another reason a cancer patient should not skip breakfast is because most chemotherapy treatment begins in the morning. If you have something in your stomach it helps you sustain the treatment with less nausea or gastrointestinal distress.

The American Heart Association found that young adults who said they ate breakfast every day were almost half as likely to be overweight as those who ate breakfast twice a week or less. Those who ate breakfast daily were also less likely to suffer from the insulin-resistance syndrome. The study drew on data collected from over 2,800 people ages twenty-five to thirty-seven. The sample was almost evenly divided between white and black Americans; whites were more than twice as likely as blacks to say they ate breakfast regularly.

The study's lead researcher, Dr. Mark Pereira of Children's Hospital in Boston, said the benefits were highest among people who ate whole-grain cereal, as opposed to refined cereal, and that eggs and bacon increased risks. For reasons that were not clear, black women did not appear to get the same protective benefits from regular breakfasts.

Shop Right

Where do you shop for foods? Do you shop in the most convenient supermarket or do you seek out fresher produce from farmers' markets or stores that carry better-quality foods? We encourage patients to shop sensibly, read labels, and search for appropriate and healthy foods and especially organic produce.

Read the list of ingredients on the label to be sure there are no trans-fatty acids (usually listed as hydrogenated or partially hydrogenated oils), artificial colors, and other undesirable products. And be sure to look at the list of grams of various nutrients, such as fiber, sugar, and sodium.

When Eating Out

We all like the occasional pizza or burger but many people seem to exist on this type of food. With little interest in food, cancer patients just do what is convenient and go to their local Pizza Hut or McDonald's on a regular basis. While you should try to limit your consumption of fast foods, you can occasionally eat in restaurants—even take-out food—without sacrificing your healthful eating goals. For example, choose the dishes that offer the freshest foods prepared in the simplest way. Avoid dishes that are fried or come with lots of sauces. These frequently contain hidden ingredients such as trans fats and prepared industrial cooking ingredients that are high in calories, sugar, and fats. Ask lots of questions of the waitstaff before you order. In good restaurants (in all price ranges) the staff should be knowledgeable and friendly and willing to tell you how the food is prepared.

In 2003, under the sponsorship and encouragement of the Breast Cancer Alliance in Greenwich, Connecticut, my office began a cooperative effort with a group of restaurants in Fairfield County in Connecticut and Westchester County in New York. Our goal was to create a series of healthy and tasty Mediterranean-style dishes with ingredients known to promote good health as well as having benefits in reducing breast cancer risk and enhancing the life of breast cancer survivors. We want to demonstrate how people can eat in fine restaurants without compromising either the quality of their dining experience or the health-giving benefits of their diet.

The menu includes dishes such as mixed organic salad with balsamic lemon vinaigrette, vegetable and lentil soup with toasted pine nuts and lemon oil, and grilled king salmon with butternut squash, broccoli rabe, and balsamic vinegar.

The Breast Cancer Alliance is a national organization but because they are based in the East, this program started here. However, they are hoping to make this a national program with restaurants all over the country offering meals that promote good health and cancer prevention.

Try a Group Nutrition Program

During treatment, cancer patients in my practice meet monthly for ninety minutes with the nutritionist, doctor, and oncology nurse. This group nutrition program offers guidelines about why weight is so important, the nature of chemotherapy-induced weight gain, risks of obesity and cancer, such as recurrence, additional cancers, and other diseases. The group setting is beneficial because patients can exchange ideas. For example, several patients who lived in the same region of the state set up a shopping schedule so that every few days one of them would be responsible for buying produce for all of them at an organic farmer's market. They were able to work this out with their chemotherapy treatment schedules so that the person doing the shopping was several days out from a treatment and would be feeling well enough.

To find a group nutrition program, contact your local cancer organization. If one does not exist in your area, encourage your cancer hospital to begin one. You might want to volunteer to set this up yourself, perhaps with the help of other cancer patients at the center or in your neighborhood.

YOUR DIETARY PLAN should not end once your cancer treatment is over. It should only be revised for life without treatment. You should have a complete workup again complete with metabolic profile, repeating all tests, so you can create a dietary plan to stick with for the rest of your life. If your oncologist is not interested or doesn't have the time to help you do this, ask if he or she can recommend a well-trained nutritionist.

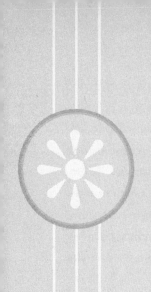

CHAPTER 6

Bad Carbs, Good Carbs: Knowing the Difference

YES, YOU DO NEED to eat carbohydrates. I don't care what fad diets claim. Carbohydrates provide nutrients, fiber, and minerals that are essential. However, most people don't really understand the difference between carbohydrates from fruit, vegetables, and whole grains and those from processed and refined foods and sugars. The wrong carbs are the critical component of what's driving the metabolic syndrome. The more you eat of these wrong carbs, the more you crave because all that free-flowing sugar is wreaking havoc on your body's insulin production.

We are a nation of sugar junkies. The United States uses more sugar than any other country in the world. The French actually add more sugar to the wine they export to the United States. The obesity epidemic in America can be blamed on our overindulgence in refined carbohydrates such as starches and sugar, which cause a spike in blood sugar. This chronic high blood sugar, combined with inactivity and stress, is a prescription for illness and death.

After the advent of agriculture, we grew increasingly dependent on fewer major food sources and were subject to periodic food shortages in times of famine. Only in the recent postindustrial era, in the face of abundant year-round, calorie-dense, nutrient-poor diets typical of Western societies, have we seen increased weight, diabetes, and heart disease. These are inevitable consequences. And so is cancer. This is now evident in underdeveloped countries undergoing transition to more Western lifestyles.

While overweight Americans are rushing to the newly popular low-carb diets, they are unwittingly omitting all carbs, rather than only the bad carbs. Low-carb products are appearing on shelves faster than we can read the labels.

Refined and Complex Carbohydrates

You need to carefully distinguish between simple and refined carbs (bad) and complex carbs (good).

* Simple carbohydrates are refined sugars and grains that we find in white bread, white rice, most pastries, and baked goods like cookies. They are also found in honey, corn syrup, and high-fructose fruits such as raisins and other dried fruit, and some melons.
* Complex carbohydrates are natural, nonprocessed plant foods—fruit or vegetables, especially legumes, and whole grains such as whole-wheat bread and oatmeal.

Refined sugar and starches or anything made from white flour are absorbed quickly into the blood and cause a spike of blood sugar and a surge of insulin within minutes. On the other hand, the longer it takes the carbohydrates to be digested—as in the case of complex carbohydrates like most vegetables and whole grains—the lesser the impact on blood sugar and insulin and the healthier the food.

Complex carbohydrates are frequently rich in fiber as well as micronutrients and contribute to the plant-based diet that is linked with weight loss and improved insulin sensitivity. Many studies have confirmed this effect. The Harvard Medical School and Children's Hospital in Boston assessed whole-grain versus refined carbohydrates in overweight and insulin-resistant adults. After a six-week dietary period, those who ate a whole-grain diet had lower insulin in the blood and a significant improvement in insulin sensitivity in contrast to those on the refined carbohydrate diet.

The CARDIA study (Coronary Artery Risk Development in Young Adults) followed 2,909 healthy adults ages eighteen to thirty for ten years. Those who ate more fiber had lower body weight, lower waist-hip ratio, and lower insulin level. This confirmed the crucial role of fiber-containing foods in limiting both obesity and the resulting insulin-resistant state.

The Glycemic Index

Many diet books are designed around the glycemic index, a ranking of how specific carbohydrate-containing foods, when eaten alone, affect the blood sugar levels. The glycemic response reflects the rise in blood sugar that occurs two hours after a 50-gram carbohydrate meal. A high glycemic index reflects a rapid though short rise in blood glucose often accompanied by a high insulin secretion in response. A low glycemic index food produces a more sustained but lower glucose rise. This is often accompanied by a reduced insulin peak response.

The index was conceived as an attempt to help diabetics gauge their dietary intake. Proponents for the index argue that foods that raise blood sugar quickly, those with a high GI ranking, such as refined carbohydrates, stimulate hunger and increase insulin. As a result, they promote the storage of fat and reduce the body's ability to burn fat. Critics maintain it is only a reference tool and has many limitations. It cannot account for the kind of complexities that may occur outside of a clinical lab setting. Many studies, however, do suggest that high glycemic index foods typical of Western diets contribute to the epidemic of obesity and insulin resistance.

If you are trying to lose weight and reduce insulin levels, then you want to eat foods with a low glycemic index. Foods in the medium range won't necessarily hurt you but they won't create any change either. Foods in the high range are the quickest to convert to sugar and therefore act to add weight and increase insulin levels. Some foods, while good for you in other ways, should be avoided if you are trying to lose weight and reduce insulin resistance. For example, watermelon is packed with vitamins and nutrients such as lycopene, but it is a high glycemic food, so should be eaten in limited quantities.

Hidden Carbs

Sucrose as well as that notorious concentrated carbohydrate corn syrup is hidden in processed foods of all kinds. Soft drinks and juices with such additives have been blamed in the rising risk of childhood obesity. While many people drink sugar-free or diet sodas, they may not know the risks there either. Aspartame, the sweetener used in Equal, may have an effect on behavior and the nervous system function. Sucralose, the sweetener found in Splenda, is made with real sugar, so it is not as harmful as some artificial sweeteners. The FDA tried to ban saccharin, which is found in Sweet'N Low, several years ago after animal testing showed that in large amounts it caused bladder cancer, but the strong industry lobbies caused them to overturn their efforts.

Plant Food and Fiber

There are two types of fiber: soluble and insoluble. Soluble is the type of fiber found in cooked oatmeal and legumes. This is a gelatinous substance that is known to help rid the body of cholesterol by sticking to it and carrying it out of the body. Insoluble fiber is the part of the food that is not absorbed: the chaff of the grain, the strings, skins, and seeds of vegetables and fruits. This fiber pulls other wastes and toxins along as it passes through the gut undigested.

There have been many studies on fiber and colon cancer risk, but few on other types of cancer. And while the debate continues on whether lack of fiber causes colon cancer, it is more important to understand that fiber reduces the metabolic syndrome, and this has very much to do with cancer. It may not be the fiber itself, but rather the ability of fiber to limit obesity and insulin resistance that is important.

The Colon Cancer Controversy

First, let's settle the controversy about fiber and colon cancer. It's long been assumed that dietary fiber helps prevent colon cancer. Early international studies in populations with high fiber intake show a reduced risk of colon cancer. An increase in fiber increases fecal water and dilutes carcinogens. This reduces transit time of stool passing through the colon. This in turn reduces exposure of the colonic cell to any carcinogen present. In addition, fiber may impact on metabolism of short-chain fatty acids, again a speculative explanation for the role of fiber in colon cancer.

However, despite much of this experimental and epidemiologic support, recent studies have now called in question the importance of fiber in colon carcinogenesis. Two very large polyp prevention studies in the United States, using high-fiber diets in people with previous polyps, showed no impact on the development of further polyp formation. This is the classic example of missing the forest for the trees. In fact, most people who eat lots of vegetable fiber are not obese. Not only that, high fiber intake is linked to a reduction in insulin resistance. Indeed, this may be the true mechanism in which fiber works. Taking people who remain on the same lifestyle with a high-fat diet, excessive weight, and little exercise and adding fiber will do nothing to blunt the insulin resistance that is linked to progression of this process.

The largest scientific study ever to investigate the links between diet and cancer risk strongly support a role for dietary fiber in the prevention of colon cancer. The American Institute for Cancer Research and the World Cancer Research Fund International in May 2003 expressed hope that the new findings will clarify a controversial issue. Researchers tracked the diets of 519,978 people in ten European countries for an average of four and a half years. They found that those who ate the most fiber had their risk of colon cancer reduced by 40 percent, compared with those who ate the least fiber. The study focused strictly on dietary fiber and did not investigate the effect of fiber supplements.

An American study used a different method but reached the same conclusion. They compared 33,917 people without colon cancer with 3,591 people who had had at least one polyp. Those who ate the most fiber had their risk of polyps reduced by 20 percent compared to those who ate the least.

Several recent fiber studies have looked at whether or not fiber can prevent colon polyps in people who had had them before. Men with a history of colon cancer were given high-fiber, low-fat diets and followed for over four years. There was no difference in the incidence of colon adenomas, including large or more advanced cancers. Several other studies came to the same conclusion. In other words, it is not the fiber itself but rather the ability of fiber to limit obesity and insulin resistance that is the explanation.

A Special Diet for Colon Cancer Patients

I give my colon cancer patients a special diet, whether they are overweight or not, because there are some nutrients and fiber that are especially important in this cancer. (Unfortunately, fiber has not been as widely studied in other cancers.)

Colon cancer patients should limit protein to fish and chicken without skin. Don't eat grilled red meat more than once a week because during the digestive process, the char on the meat forms a carcinogen. This is especially useful for prevention and for survivors who want to lower their risk of recurrence.

Eat six to ten servings of fruits and vegetables a day, including high-fiber produce. Make fruits and vegetables the major portion of your meals, with meat as a side dish.

Take a calcium supplement of 1,200 to 1,500 grams a day, and 600 to 800 units of vitamin D. The latter is especially important if you live in northern regions, where there is less sunlight. (See page 131 for the most effective calcium supplements.) Also take 200 micrograms a day of selenium.

Avoid excessive folate (folic acid) supplements. Once you have colon cancer, folate may enhance the growth of undetected cancer cells. (It is preventive in very early stages of premalignancy.) Folate (400 micrograms or less a day) should only be used for patients who cannot eat enough folate in their diet.

Eat plain yogurt daily, not only for the important milk proteins, but to maintain healthy bowel flora.

Fiber Reduces Insulin Resistance

The debate about fiber will continue, but fiber is clearly needed for the digestive system to work properly. It produces more bulky stools and thus faster transit time for stools through the colon. Not only does this mean less constipation, which is important for health as well as for patients who are on chemotherapy where constipation can be a problem, it also may reduce the exposure of the colon wall to toxic compounds related to cancer risk.

However, its real benefit may be that as a component of a healthy diet rich in fruits and vegetables, it contributes to a reduction in insulin resistance. Indeed, in the insulin-resistance atherosclerosis study, evaluating 978 middle-aged adults with normal or impaired glucose tolerance, those people on a whole-grain diet with dark breads and high-fiber cereal showed significant reduction in fasting insulin and improvement overall in insulin sensitivity. This again confirms that higher intakes of whole grains are associated with improvement in insulin sensitivity and a reduction in insulin resistance consistent with this potential effect.

Bread, Pasta, and Other High-Starch Carbohydrates

Grains provide necessary vitamins, especially B vitamins, and minerals as well as fiber, so you need them. While high levels of pasta can be high glycemic, leading to a higher insulin production and higher body fat, both high-quality whole-wheat and spinach pasta may help you avoid this. Whole-wheat breads are preferred to white breads.

Sugars, including powdered and cane, as well as honey should be limited. All manufactured products containing corn syrup and high-fructose syrup are dangerously high in concentrated sugar and boost insulin and weight.

Prepackaged products containing processed, refined carbs are high in fat and calories and low in fiber. They are high on the glycemic index and also high in trans-fatty acids (see the next chapter) to give them a long shelf life. On the lists at the end of the chapter you will find the good and bad carbs, but remember the stress factor. Too much restriction in a diet may cause stress, so if you love mashed potatoes, then have a small portion once in a while. Potatoes are high on the glycemic index, but they also possess many vitamins and minerals.

Vegetables: The Best Carbs

Fresh vegetables are low in calories. They add variety and flavor to your diet and provide fiber, vitamins, phytonutrients, antioxidants, and anti-inflammatories. They fill you up without making you fat. Most American diets are very low in vegetables. A typical dinner meal is usually planned around a meat or fish dish, then supplemented with a potato or pasta and only one green or yellow vegetable. The best way to change this pattern is to plan your meal around the vegetables. Have a salad plus two other veggies and make the meat a small percentage of the meal. For example, a vegetable stir-fry using olive oil may contain several vegetables and a small amount of meat.

As mentioned earlier, it's been proven that most people do not eat enough fruit and vegetables every day to get all the nutrients and fiber they need. For example, the American Institute for Cancer Research (AICR) has been suggesting that the way to reduce the risk of cancer is to keep weight down, exercise regularly, and eat five or more servings of vegetables and fruit a day. In a thirteen-year AICR study led by the Mayo Clinic College of Medicine, the hardest thing for the survey participants to do was comply with the fruit and vegetable criteria. Only 11 percent of the thirty thousand postmenopausal women surveyed complied.

Vegetables should not be overcooked and are preferable fresh and not canned. If you cannot get fresh, then frozen is best. Vegetables are usually frozen right after harvesting so they retain more of their nutrients than canned.

In addition to fiber, whole grains, vegetables, and fruit contribute a variety of vitamins and minerals, particularly folate, which has been well documented in reducing colon cancer.

And while no one vegetable is going to cure cancer, you should be aware of some that are especially beneficial. Include these frequently.

Cruciferous Vegetables

Cruciferous vegetables have a well-deserved reputation for cancer prevention. Broccoli, cauliflower, Brussels sprouts, kale, and arugula are all valuable. There are several reasons these should form an important part of your diet.

* They are rich in vitamins, including folic acid, and the carotenoids (lutein, beta and alpha carotene, zeoxanthine). Foods rich in carotenoids are linked to a lower risk of breast cancer, particularly for women prior to menopause and with a family history.
* They have abundant and healthy fiber content that will help in weight control as well as limit the development of insulin resistance, which is associated with poorer outcomes with breast cancer and potentially, a higher risk of getting cancer.
* Most cruciferous vegetables, particularly broccoli, contain an important phytonutrient—isothiocyanates—that enhances the metabolism of carcinogens, reducing their levels in the

body. They also may alter the metabolism of estrogen in the body, changing it to a much less potent metabolite with a reduced breast cancer stimulatory effect.

Tomatoes

Tomatoes, a mainstay of the Mediterranean diet, contain a pigment called lycopene that is responsible for their red color. This is a powerful antioxidant. Tomatoes in all their forms—canned stewed tomatoes, tomato soup, tomato juice, and even ketchup—are major sources of lycopene. Tomatoes are also high in vitamin C. Their rich nutrients are released when cooked in olive oil. While likely beneficial in protecting against breast cancer, lycopene has been particularly linked to a lower risk of prostate cancer. In Greece, the foods most associated with a low level of insulin-like growth factor 1, a potent cancer cell stimulus for most forms of cancer, were lycopene-rich foods. Thus, tomatoes are an important part of a good diet.

A Harvard study concluded that men who ate lycopene-rich diets had a much lower risk of developing certain cancers, especially prostate. Women with high lycopene levels had less risk of precancerous signs of cervical cancer.

Another "red" plant food is watermelon, also rich in lycopene as well as vitamins A, B, and C, and potassium. However, it is high on the glycemic index and converts to sugar quickly in the body. If you are insulin resistant, eat this fruit sparingly.

The Allium Family

Any member of the allium family of vegetables has potent phytonutrients that have been shown to add to the cancer protection effect of a high vegetable diet. These include garlic, onions, leeks, asparagus, and scallions. They contain a variety of sulfur-containing compounds that are crucial in both antioxidant and anticarcinogen pathways. There is more quercetin—an antioxidant—in onions than there is in tea and apples. Onions are also a great source of vitamin C, folic acid, and fiber, all important to maintaining health.

Mushrooms

Mushrooms have many valuable nutrients. In fact, interest in the immune-stimulating components of both shiitake and maitake mushrooms has led to the use of mushroom extracts for cancer treatment. As a food they are an important part of the total vegetable content.

Carrots

Beta-carotene is an orange pigment isolated from carrots 150 years ago. It is found concentrated in deep orange and green vegetables (the green chlorophyll covers up the orange pigment). Beta-carotene is an antioxidant that has been much discussed in connection with lung cancer. The evidence is conflicting but further research is being done to see if it has a protective effect. In the meantime, you need orange and yellow vegetables like carrots for their antioxidant value.

Herbs and Seasonings

Keep in mind that seasonings are taken from plants and contain nutrients. They are rich in phytochemicals that protect against disease. Naturopathic medicine and most traditional medicines such as ayurveda, Native American, and Chinese have emphasized the healing properties of common herbs. However, we know them primarily for their role as flavorings. Useful herbs with anticancer properties include turmeric, rosemary, ginger, and fennel.

* Oregano contains quercetin, a strong antioxidant that is protective against cancers. According to a U.S. Department of Agriculture study, oregano has the most antioxidant of all the herbs studied. It also has forty-two times more than apples, thirty times more than potatoes, and twelve times more than oranges.

* Turmeric is yellow because of curcumin, which slows the proliferation of prostate cancer cells and has potent anti-inflammatory properties as well.

* Fresh ginger has gingerol and when dried, zingerone. Both are antioxidant and anti-inflammatory. And ginger, according to many studies, may enhance the antinausea effects of conventional medications for people on chemotherapy.

Beans and Legumes

Legumes and beans (known as pulses) play an important role in the traditional diets of many regions throughout the world. However, in Western countries, beans play a less important dietary role despite being low in fat and excellent sources of protein, dietary fiber, vitamin B, iron, calcium, and a variety of micronutrients and phytochemicals. The soluble fiber in legumes helps to control blood cholesterol and blood sugar levels. Pulses have the right percentage of protein and carbohydrates. We only need a small amount for good health. Try to eat one serving of legumes, such as kidney beans, butter beans, lima beans, lentils, or chickpeas, every day.

A 2002 report by the Metabolic Research Group at the University of Kentucky found that dried beans reduce cholesterol levels and prevent heart disease because they have high levels of soluble fiber. Beans are low on the glycemic index. And despite being fairly high in calories, eating beans can also help you lose weight because they stimulate hormones that decrease hunger. In addition, they may help you live longer, according to a recent Australian study that found a positive correlation between eating dried beans and longevity.

Soy

Soybeans are unique among the legumes because they are a concentrated source of isoflavones, which have weak estrogenic properties. Foods made with soy have received considerable attention for their potential role in preventing and treating cancer and osteoporosis. Isoflavones are powerful antioxidants. Genistein is the most potent one found in soy, followed by daidzein.

The lower breast cancer mortality rates in Asian countries and the putative antiestrogen effects of isoflavones have fueled speculation that eating soy reduces breast cancer risk. Thus, many women are confused about soy. To add to the confusion, the timing of exposure to soy may play a role in breast cancer in Asia. Young women who are exposed to phytoestrogen compounds such as soy before puberty may actually have an early and more rapid maturation of their breast tissue, making them less sensitive to the development of breast cancer as adults. Thus, the timing of exposure may also be a critical reason why soy in Asian populations has benefits in terms of breast cancer reduction. Conversely, higher levels of soy in women past puberty, particularly in middle age, may have the opposite effect in stimulating breast cell growth. While Asian women have a high soy intake and a low breast cancer rate, it is likely that many other factors are also at play. In fact, women who take soy powder supplements or soy isoflavones often enriched in the soy components, such as genistein and daidzein, may be placing themselves at higher risk. At very high levels, these compounds have a mild estrogen-stimulating effect. In several studies, there is evidence they may interfere with the anti–breast cancer drug tamoxifen.

However, women who consume foods with soy, including tofu and miso, are at no risk and may benefit from many other healthy nutrients as well as high-quality protein. The key is dietary diversity.

The available data suggesting that, in contrast to breast cancer, soy or isoflavones may reduce the risk of prostate cancer are more encouraging.

Helpful Hints

Beans are convenient to use. For example, lentils need no soaking and canned varieties are ready to use. Mix lentils with minced turkey or chicken for spaghetti Bolognese or lasagna. Mix some kidney beans with minced chicken or turkey for a tasty chili con carne. Make a curry with chicken and chickpeas, or a stew or casserole of lean lamb and beans. Make a dip, such as hummus. Try black bean or lentil soup, or make a variety of salsas with beans, tomatoes, onions, and cilantro.

Fruit

Fruits contain fiber, vitamins, and minerals. Eat them fresh whenever you can. Otherwise dried or frozen fruit is good, or canned fruit that does not contain sugar syrups. A serving size for fresh fruit is one medium piece, about the size of a baseball.

Citrus fruits such as oranges, grapefruit, lemons, and limes contain many natural substances that appear to be important in disease protection, such as carotenoids, flavonoids, and others. Together, these phytochemicals act more powerfully than if they were given separately. It's always better to eat the fruit whole in its natural form, as some of the potency is lost when the juice is extracted and most often sugar is added.

Red Wine

Red wine is made of a fruit rich not only in polyphenols but also in other important phytonutrients, including resveratrol. This nutrient has been suggested to reduce aging and there is ongoing research trying to isolate the crucial and stable resveratrol component.

But alcohol presents a problem. There is an increased risk of breast cancer with increasing alcohol intake in women. However, if you get a rich supply of foods with a high folate content (green leafy vegetables, orange juice) it may negate this adverse affect. Because wine (particularly red wine) is an important and healthy component of the Mediterranean diet and is also enriched with healthy polyphenols (as is olive oil), having a healthy salad and lots of cruciferous vegetables will reduce the guilt and increase the benefits of a glass of pinot noir or cabernet sauvignon.

Chocolate

Chocolate comes from the cocoa plant so perhaps it should be considered a fruit. However, chocolate, as we know it, is a candy or dessert. It also contains antioxidants and flavonoids. In modest amounts, dark chocolate has polyphenols and may lower cholesterol ever so slightly. Women undergoing chemotherapy often crave chocolate, and a small amount may satisfy this craving. Dark chocolate is better for you because it has less sugar than milk chocolate.

Grains and Starches to Choose

All-Bran cereal

Barley (pearled and cracked but not rolled)

Brown rice

Buckwheat

Egg fettuccine, linguine, and spaghetti

Oat bran cereal high in protein and fiber

Oatmeal (traditional, not instant)

Rye (whole kernels)

Semolina

Uncle Sam dry cereal

Vita Wheat Crisp

Wasa Crackers

Whole-wheat bread with at least 3 grams of fiber

Whole-wheat pita

Whole-wheat tortilla

Whole-wheat waffle (reduced fat, high protein)

Grains and Starches to Avoid

Bagels

Granola

Grape-Nuts cereal

Instant oatmeal

Muffins

Pastry

Potato chips

Pretzels

Puffed cereals

Pumpernickel bread

Rice cereal

Rye bread

Tortilla chips

White bread

White-flour pasta

White rice

Vegetables to Choose

The serving size for raw leafy vegetables is one cup—that equals the size of a baseball or the fist of an average adult. The serving size for chopped raw vegetable is half a cup—the size of half a baseball or a rounded handful for an average adult. Cooked vegetables are also half a cup. However, keep in mind that you can eat more than one serving size if you are hungry.

Artichoke hearts

Arugula

Asparagus

Bamboo shoots

Beans (green, wax, Italian, haricots verts)

Broccoli

Brussels sprouts

Cabbage (red, green, Chinese)

Carrots

Cauliflower

Celery

Chives

Cucumber

Eggplant

Endive

Garlic

Kohlrabi

Leeks

Lettuce (except iceberg) and micro-greens

Mushrooms

Okra

Onions (all varieties, including scallions, shallots, leeks)

Peppers (all varieties)

Snow peas

Spinach

Squash (zucchini, summer, yellow, spaghetti)

Tomatoes (fresh, juice, canned or cooked)

Turnips

Water chestnuts

Watercress

Vegetables to Limit

These vegetables, with their high starch and sugar content, are high on the glycemic index. Also, avoid any vegetables that are battered and deep-fried or cooked with cream sauce.

Beets

Corn

Pumpkin

Fruit to Choose

Apples

Applesauce, unsweetened

Apricots

Berries (except strawberries)

Cantaloupe

Cherries

Figs

Grapefruit

Guavas

Honeydew melons

Kiwifruit

Lychees

Mandarin orange

Mangoes

Nectarines

Oranges

Papayas

Peaches

Pears

Pineapples

Plums

Fruit to Limit

Bananas

Canned fruits packed in heavy syrup

Dates

Grapes

Raisins

Strawberries

Watermelon

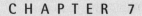

CHAPTER 7

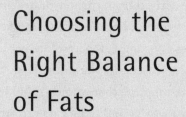

Choosing the Right Balance of Fats

FATS ARE NECESSARY for sustaining life. Every cell in our body would wither and die without fats. Some fat is needed to make cancer drugs work better. But fats can also clog our arteries and cause inflammation, as well as do other damage. Many people don't understand the difference between good and bad fats, nor do they realize how much fat they need in their daily diet.

In the 1990s we were told to eat less fat. As a result, many of us consumed more carbohydrates. "Low fat" became a marketing term used to exploit the public's interest in healthy foods and lower weight. Unwittingly, the outcome may have been the opposite of what was intended. These so-called low-fat cookies and other manufactured products substituted higher levels of refined carbohydrates. If anyone read the package labels they would notice that many of these low-fat or no-fat products had more calories than their fat-containing partners. Once again, we are drawn into an all-or-nothing diet attitude rather than focusing on balanced healthy nutrition and sustainable diet pattern.

In the recent U.S. Centers for Disease Control review of changes in food over the last thirty years, there has been an increase in the percentage of energy derived from carbohydrates and a decline in the percent of energy from fat. Because of the significant overall increase in total calories consumed, the absolute per capita fat consumption has in fact increased, despite eating less.

There was an old assumption that women should avoid high-fat foods to prevent breast cancer and reduce its growth. This is now felt to be only important in young adolescent women who eat higher-fat diets. Thus, our meals do not need to be without fat but rather directed to healthy fats, in modest proportions to limit total calorie content and with a diverse mix of nutrients.

Bad Fats

Saturated fats are mainly animal fats from meat and dairy products. They are also found in tropical oils such as palm oil (used in junk food). They raise total cholesterol, making them only marginally less risky than trans-fatty acids (see below). High saturated fats also promote higher insulin resistance. Butter, lard, solid margarine, mayonnaise, commercial salad dressings, and fat on meat—this is all saturated fat. So are most kinds of cheese and regular milk. (The next chapter about protein will provide more information on animal fats.)

Trans-fatty acids are produced when liquid oils are converted into saturated—or solid fats—by adding hydrogen atoms to them, as in shortening. These hydrogenated fats—made for fried fast foods such as French fries and commercial foods like baked pas-

Moderate Fat Diet for Breast Cancer Patients

In advising my breast cancer patients to eat a moderate fat diet, I ask them to limit red meat to once a week and eat cold-water fish such as wild salmon, sardines, and trout three times a week. Eat poultry without the skin and stick with nonfat dairy products. Use olive or canola oil in cooking and avoid corn-oil-based margarines. Never eat foods containing trans-fatty acids.

Enjoy unlimited fresh fruits and vegetables, especially the cruciferous ones such as broccoli, Brussels sprouts, and cabbage. Avoid fruit juices that are not 100 percent natural, or those with added artificial ingredients, corn syrup, fructose or honey. Eat whole-grain breads, cereals, and pastas. Use soy only as a food, not a supplement. Avoid salted or pickled foods as well as candy, and artificial sweeteners, except for stevia.

Drink a limited amount of decaffeinated coffee, but do drink two cups of tea a day—black or green. Alcohol increases breast cell growth, so avoid it.

Supplements include one high-quality multivitamin/mineral tablet daily; one 1,000 mg capsule of omega-3 (EPA/DHA) with meals; one capsule (no greater than 200 IUs) a day of mixed tocopherol/tocotrienol with the largest meal; selenium (200 mcg/a day); folate (400 mg daily). I prescribe CoQ_{10} (100 mg a day) to my patients who are taking Adriamycin or epirubicin. Probiotics are also prescribed (1 capsule daily) during chemotherapy to restore bowel flora.

When you take selenium and other vitamins, always deduct the amount you would get from your multivitamin. Don't take megadoses of vitamins. Use no more than 500 mgs of vitamin C, 200 IU of vitamin E, 800 mg of folate. Also avoid intravenous vitamin therapy while on chemotherapy.

tries, cookies, and crackers to extend shelf life—pack a double punch. They increase the bad cholesterol (LDL), which clogs arteries. And they fail to raise the good cholesterol (HDL), which cleanses arteries. Your body does not know how to break them down and use them correctly. Normal fats are pliable (even on your brain surfaces) and soft, but trans fats are stiff and can build up in the lining of your blood vessels and on your brain surfaces. Trans fats have been closely linked to inflammation, raising the risk of both heart disease and cancer through this effect. They are clearly linked to higher risks of insulin resistance and the metabolic syndrome.

Never eat these fats. Read labels and don't use products that list *hydrogenated* or *partially hydrogenated* oils or vegetable shortening. Keep in mind that the higher up on the list of ingredients, the larger the proportion of this type of fat is in the food. Fast foods and cheaper foods tend to include these fats to stabilize ingredients.

The government now requires fast-food producers to list the use of trans-fatty acids. McDonald's pledged to reduce its use of these fats in their products. Some brands of bread, crackers, and snack foods now say "No trans fats" on their package labels. Fleischmann's original and unsalted margarines are now produced without trans fats. More food producers will join in eventually. In the meantime, read the labels carefully.

Good Fats

Monounsaturated fats, typified by olive oil, predominate in the Mediterranean diet and are healthy. (Remember those long-lived Spanish women.) These fats, when substituted for saturated fats, help lower bad cholesterol (LDL). In addition, dietary patterns with significant monounsaturated fats tend to be associated with reduction in cancer risk as well as a reduction in overall mortality. Olive oil is an excellent ingredient, rich in monounsaturated fat, and extra-virgin olive oil is loaded with polyphenols, very important antioxidants with benefits for both the heart and cancer. According to recent research, the highest levels of hydroxytyrosol, a powerful antioxidant that reduces inflammation and counteracts oxidative stress, is found in some Spanish olive oils.

Polyunsaturated fats are termed essential dietary fats because the body may not be able to synthesize them. They are crucial for growth and normal cellular function. There are two types. Omega-6 (N-6) is abundant in most vegetable oils. Omega-3 (N-3) occurs in vegetable oils including canola and flaxseed, and most particularly cold-water fish and walnuts. Consuming more polyunsaturated than saturated fat is linked to a lower risk of type 2 diabetes and insulin resistance.

Essential Fatty Acids

While many Americans have cut back on fat, there still remains an unhealthy amount in many diets. Researchers at the American Institute for Cancer Research expressed concern that American diets are overloaded with omega-6 fats and deficient in omega-3 fats, and this is linked to cancer risk.

Higher omega-3 fats and lower omega-6 fats are typical of both the Mediterranean and Paleolithic diets. In contrast, the typical Western diet is unbalanced, with a much higher ratio of omega-6 to omega-3 fat because of our increasing penchant for processed and refined foods. In some American diets, the ratio of omega-6 to omega-3 is as high as 15 to 1, rather than the healthy ratio of 4 to 1 or even 2 to 1 found in countries where a traditional plant-based diet is consumed. The omega-3 and omega-6 ratio can be adjusted by using only olive or canola oil and by avoiding the use of corn oil–based products

Both omega-6 and omega-3 fats are metabolized similarly in the body, and because their molecular structure is so similar, they compete for many of the same enzymes. However, once they hook up with an enzyme, they behave differently. The molecules that arise when omega-3 fatty acids are metabolized provide a range of potential anticancer benefits. They show the ability to reduce the production of other cancer-promoting enzymes, increase the rate at which cancer cells die, and help keep cancer cells from forming the new blood vessels (angiogenesis) needed for them to grow. On the other hand, when the omega-6 fats pair with an enzyme, the resulting molecules can promote inflammation, spur cells to multiply, and decrease cancer cell death. While there is a role for omega-6 fats, when they are way out of a healthy proportion they cut off the protective benefits of the omega-3s.

* Omega-6 fats are found in vegetable oils such as corn, safflower, sunflower, and soybean. These oils are often used in processed snacks, baked products, and commercial salad dressing.

* Omega-3 fats are found mostly in fish like salmon, sardines, trout, and herring. Smaller amounts are found in canola oil, flaxseed, green leafy vegetables, and walnuts. The best seafood sources are cold-water fish. The best plant-food sources are flaxseed and flaxseed oil, canola oil, walnuts, soybeans, wheat germ, and green leafy vegetables such as spinach, kale, leeks, and broccoli.

We have known for years that a high ratio of omega-6 to omega-3 fatty acids has been linked to heart disease, but now we know it is a link in cancer, too. When omega fats are in balance, the risk for breast, prostate, and colon cancers is lower. So is the risk for inflammatory conditions such as arthritis. Omega-3 fats contribute to the improvement in the nutritional and immune status of patients with advanced cancer and in some cases a longer survival.

Adding omega-3 fatty acids to the diet of mice can actually reduce the occurrence of tumors and slow tumor growth. Omega-3 fats also potentially help chemotherapy drugs work more effectively and reduce the side effects of treatment. Other research is looking at how a particular omega-3 fatty acid (docosahexanoic acid, or DHA) interferes with a specific protein that is critical for tumor formation in the colon.

Reducing the Inflammatory State

Omega-3 fatty acids, such as fish oils, reduce the inflammatory effect of the metabolic syndrome and help prevent insulin resistance. In contrast, diets rich in omega-6 fats, particularly the corn oil used in fast foods, have been shown to increase inflammation and may enhance tumor growth and development.

The American Institute for Cancer Research is the latest to announce its support of the U.S. Food and Drug Administration decision to permit nutrient content claims for foods rich in omega-3s, given a link between omega-3s and reduced risk of some cancers. This supports the calls by the Department of Agriculture, the American Heart Association, and the National Academy of Sciences for increased consumption of omega-3s, a critical nutrient in the American diet.

Nuts and Seeds

Walnuts are unique in that they have the perfect balance of omega-6 and omega-3 polyunsaturated fatty acids, a ratio of 4 to 1. Walnuts also work as an anti-inflammatory.

While nuts contain 70 to 80 percent fat, most fatty acids in nuts are *unsaturated,* which may be beneficial for glucose and insulin sensitivity. Nuts are rich in minerals like iron and magnesium. They have also been shown to be beneficial in reducing cardiovascular risk.

One ounce of walnuts fulfills the daily requirement of 2.5 grams of omega-3 fatty acids. It's an easy way to get that essential nutrient. With news about toxins in certain marine sources of omega-3s, the American Institute for Cancer Research recommends walnuts as an alternative beneficial source of this essential nutrient.

Eat nuts in moderation. One-third of a cup or a level handful for the average adult is enough. Avoid peanut butter unless it is made without trans fats or hydrogenated oil.

Flaxseeds can be added to salads and cereals, but should be freshly ground to release their valuable contents (DHA, a healthy form of omega-3). The flax also contains lignans, which favorably reduce the more potent forms of estrogen in the system, limiting breast cancer cell stimulation. DHA also inhibits a potent stimulator of breast cancer cell growth, IGF-1, that is linked to obesity and high insulin levels.

See below for the best sources of omega-3 fatty acids. In the next chapter you will find the best seafood sources. In addition, the chapter on supplements has more information on this important anti-inflammatory.

Fats to Choose

Almonds

Canola oil

Cashews

Mayonnaise made with canola oil

Olive oil

Peanuts (avoid peanut butter made with trans fats)

Pecans

Reduced-fat salad dressing

Soft tub margarines labeled "No TFA," made with 30 to 50 percent vegetable oil

Walnuts

Fats to Avoid

Butter

Cheese (see next chapter for acceptable cheeses)

Coconut

Corn oil

Lard

Margarine (stick)

Mayonnaise (most commercial brands)

Peanut butter (unless it is organic)

Peanut oil sauces

Pistachio nuts

Salad dressings (commercial)

Shortening (hard)

Side bacon

Suet

Trans-fatty acids (TFA)

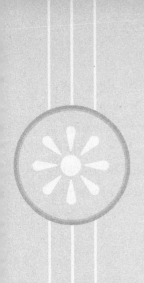

CHAPTER 8

Choosing Protein: Meat, Fish, Eggs, and Dairy Products

WE NEED PROTEIN in our diets in order to get essential vitamins and minerals. However, while meat is a good source of protein and iron, it is also a source of saturated fat and cholesterol.
Fish is a great source of protein and omega-3 fatty acids, but can
be a source of mercury, which is toxic, as well as organic pollutants
such as PCBs. An egg is an almost perfect protein and full of nutrients but the yolks have so much cholesterol that they should be
eaten in moderation. Milk and other dairy products are made from
animal fat, but the protein and calcium they provide are essential
to health. We know, in fact, that the protein and calcium in milk
help prevent insulin resistance.

Finding the right balance of protein in a diverse diet is important. Too much protein can lead to calcium and bone loss because
it creates high phosphate levels. This may be an issue for anyone

with impaired kidney function because it limits their ability to handle the nitrogen load inherent in protein.

If you are a vegetarian, there are many alternatives for getting the proper amount of protein and minerals you would normally get from meat and fish. Legumes (including tofu from soybeans), for example, can be combined with certain low-fat dairy products to come up with the right protein combination.

Meat and Poultry

For tens of thousands of years, we ate the flesh of animals that lived on grass and vegetation and remained constantly on the move. Today, cattle are raised in pens and are fed from a common trough and hoses. Isn't it ironic that cattle have ended up with a sedentary lifestyle much like our own?

We need look no further than the mad cow scare in late 2003 to understand how flawed our entire meat production system is or how far we have come from what nature intended. We raise cattle in factories and we have flouted evolutionary rules by turning natural herbivores into heavy but often ill-nourished animals with a high-calorie diet, including antibiotics and hormones designed to make them fat, and thus, tastier.

Eat Meat in Moderation

I want my patients to rely on chicken and fish for protein and limit red meat to once or twice a week. They should also drink three glasses of low-fat or skim milk a day for the valuable protein as well as the calcium and vitamin D.

Try to find free-range or organic meat that is grown without hormones. However, not finding it doesn't mean you are at particular risk. When your diet is based on large quantities of fruits and vegetables, you lower your risk of harm from possible carcinogens in meat and poultry.

The weight of meat or fish is measured after it is cooked. A quarter of a pound (four ounces) usually shrinks to a standard three-ounce serving, about the size of a deck of cards.

✳ Skin poultry and trim fat from all meats before cooking.

✳ Use cooking methods that allow fat to drip away from the meat, such as braising, roasting, and broiling. Grilled meat generates high levels of polycyclic aromatic hydrocarbons in the char. These form when food is kept in direct flame for more than brief periods during the grilling process. In the gastrointestinal tract, bacteria may convert them to more potent cancer-causing compounds.

✳ Make stews and soups ahead of time and refrigerate. When they are cooled, remove the congealed fat from the top before you reheat the dish.

✳ When you make meat sauces or casseroles, brown the meat first. Then, discard the fat and add the meat to the other ingredients.

✳ Never cook meat with butter or solid margarines that are rich in hydrogenated fats.

What to Know about Fish

Fish is a great low-fat source of protein. Try to eat fish high in omega-3 fatty acids often. These include salmon, sardines, trout, mackerel, and Pacific oysters.

While high in omega-3 fatty acids, some of these fish pose other risks, such as mercury and high levels of pesticides. The level of pesticide residues in farm salmon is highest in Atlantic farm-raised salmon, particularly from Scotland and the Faro Islands. It is lowest in farm-raised salmon from Chile and Washington state. The safest salmon is from the Pacific Ocean. It is the food given to the salmon, not the water they are kept in, that leads to high PCB levels.

Limit farmed salmon to one or two servings a month. This is especially important for children and pregnant women. Look for wild salmon, which is usually available frozen or canned. To reduce the risk of ingesting PCBs, remove the skin and any visible fat from fish. Bake, broil, or poach fish rather than frying. Fish oil has been assessed in several studies and confirmed to be low in organic pesticide residues as well as mercury (like salmon itself), making it a safe alternative to eating salmon.

Avoid mackerel and tuna, both of which are high in mercury. Americans tend to like tuna fish sandwiches and two of these a week can contain as much as 35 micrograms of mercury, close to the 38.5 microgram weekly limit recommended by the National Academy of Sciences and the EPA. This statistic applies to white tuna; light tuna has less.

Some shellfish, such as shrimp and lobster, as well as caviar and fish roe, are high in cholesterol. However, they are safe to eat in limited amounts.

Lists at the end of the chapter compare the mercury levels and omega-3 levels for selected fish so you can make wise choices. Unfortunately, the fish with the lowest mercury levels don't always have the highest omega-3 levels. The best fish in both categories include salmon, sardines, oysters, and trout. While tuna has high omega-3 levels, it also has very high mercury levels.

Eggs

Because of the high cholesterol level in egg yolks it's a good idea to limit consumption to three eggs a week, particularly if you have elevated cholesterol or are at high risk for heart disease. However, keep in mind that many of the other foods you eat may already contain eggs, such as baked goods, pancakes, some sauces, and dressings. The reduced fat and cholesterol in Egg Beaters are okay in moderation.

Some people eat only the whites of the eggs, which are a great source of protein without the fat. You can often find "white omelettes" on restaurant menus. This is strictly a matter of taste. Some people find this a tasty solution if they mix other things into the omelette, but others say why bother.

The Role of Milk and Dairy Products

Most of us know that milk is the best source of calcium, but it may actually be the high-quality protein in milk that is important in combating cancer and the metabolic syndrome. Milk and dairy products limit weight gain in children and adults and may, in fact, enhance weight loss. They also may contribute to reduction in cancer development and improved prognosis through several important nutrients, including vitamin D, calcium, fats such as conjugated linoleic acid, and whey protein, the major protein in dairy products. Ironically, many patients often avoid eating dairy products out of misplaced concerns about whether they are good for them. Prostate cancer is the only case where we are concerned about dairy (particularly whole milk products), because of excessive calcium and saturated milk fat. Men should eat only low-fat dairy products and be sure to get adequate vitamin D. (It will also help stave off osteoporosis, which men often are unaware they can develop as they age.)

Low-fat dairy products are beneficial for their high-quality protein, high calcium, and several additional nutrients, including CLA (conjugated linoleic acid), found only in dairy products and shown to have a direct anti–breast cancer effect.

An eight-ounce glass of milk provides 30 percent of the RDA of calcium; eight ounces of yogurt provide 25 percent; and four ounces of cheese provide 80 percent. Here's the cholesterol content of milk: In one cup of whole milk there are 34 milligrams of cholesterol compared to 5 milligrams in skim milk. Milk with 2 percent fat has 22 milligrams.

Cheeses contain varying amounts of fat. Remember that vegetarian cheeses made with soy contain as many calories from fat as ordinary cheeses. Cheese can make a healthy breakfast with fruit or bread. Many low-fat spreads and cottage cheese have added tasty flavoring such as smoked salmon or pineapple. There are now numerous other low-fat choices for cheese.

Yogurt is enriched with a variety of healthy bacteria that in some studies have been linked to lower cancer rates, including breast and particularly colon cancer. For the cancer patient on treatment as well as cancer survivors, yogurt is very helpful to rebalance the bowel flora.

The Impact on Insulin Resistance

A study in the *Journal of the American Medical Association* revealed that increased dairy consumption lowers insulin resistance among overweight adults and may reduce the risk of type 2 diabetes and heart disease.

The CARDIA study of young adults showed that for every dairy product consumed in a day, there was a 21 percent decrease in risk for insulin resistance. The odds of developing the metabolic syndrome are 72 percent lower if you eat dairy products thirty-five times a week rather than ten times a week.

Meat and Poultry to Choose

Beef: round steak, rump roast, sirloin tip, lean ground or minced steak

Lamb: leg, loin, shank

Pork: tenderloin, ham, center cut, bacon, loin chops

Poultry: chicken, turkey, Cornish hens

Meat and Poultry to Avoid

Beef: fatty, marbled, and prime cut meat or hamburger

Lamb: mutton or ground

Pork: side of bacon, ham hocks, pig's feet, spare ribs, and short ribs

Poultry: duck, goose, stewing hens, commercially fried chicken

Fish with Low Mercury Levels

Eat all you want from this list.

Fish	Omega-3 levels
Catfish	Low
Clams	Low
Orange roughy	Low
Oysters (Pacific)	High

Oysters (elsewhere)	Medium
Salmon	High
Sardines	High
Shrimp	Low
Tilapia	Low

Fish with Medium Mercury Levels

It is safe to eat these fish once a week, but women in their reproductive years should limit mahimahi and red snapper (which have the highest mercury levels in this group) to once a month.

Fish	Omega-3 Level
Flounder	Medium
Mahimahi	Low
Red snapper	Low
Trout	High

Fish with High Mercury Levels

Avoid these fish. A single meal can put you over the EPA safe limit for the month.

Fish	Omega-3 Level
Amberjack	Low
Chilean sea bass	Medium

Grouper	Low
Halibut	Low
Shark	Medium
Swordfish	Medium
Tuna (fresh)	High

Dairy Products to Choose

Buttermilk (less than 1 percent fat)

Milk (skim, fat-free, 1 percent, evaporated skim)

Powdered milk (fat-free or low-fat)

Yogurt (fat-free)

Very Low-Fat and Fat-Free Cheese (0.4 to 5 percent)

Cottage cheese (fat-free and very low-fat)

Fromage frais (virtually fat-free)

Low-Fat Cheese (5 to 12 percent)

Low-fat solid cheeses such as Babybel Light, Edam, Kraft, mozzarella

Low-fat cheese spreads and soft cheeses such as Boursin Light, Laughing Cow, fromage frais, and Philadelphia

Medium-Fat Cheese (15 to 26 percent)

Austrian smoked cheese

Brie

Camembert

Cheddars (low-fat, such as Cabot)

Cream cheese such as Philadelphia Light

Edam

Feta

Goat

Grana Padano

Mozzarella

Ricotta, part skim

Dairy Products to Limit

Butter

Buttermilk

Dairy substitutes or coffee whiteners

Half and half

Heavy cream

Milk (whole, chocolate, evaporated, condensed)

Ice cream, ice milk, gelato

Sour cream

Yogurt (fruit-flavored, high-fat)

High-Fat Cheese (27 to 42 percent fat)

Boursin

Blue cheese

Cheddar, vegetarian cheddar

Cheddar cheese stick

Cheshire

Double Gloucester

Emmental

Gouda

Gruyère

Jarlsberg

Mascarpone

Parmesan

Roquefort

Roule

Stilton

Some Helpful Tips

* Use yogurt in place of sour cream or mayonnaise in salad
   dressings and sauces.
* Mix fat-free yogurt such as Total or Stonyfield Farm with
   fresh or frozen fruit for a nutritious breakfast.
* Do the same with low-fat cottage cheese.

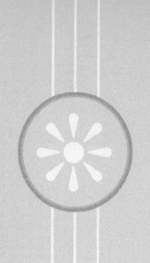

CHAPTER 9

Nutritional Supplements to Aid in Your Treatment

MOST PEOPLE at one time or another have taken nutritional supplements, often without medical guidance, and frequently from uncertain sources with limited quality assurance and little consideration of risks and benefits.

The role of supplements is just that, as a "supplement" to a good diet, not a substitute. The best source of nutrients is from appropriate food sources. Nature provides foods with an abundance of micronutrients in combinations and in forms most effective in disease prevention and for general health. Many benefits derived from foods, particularly a variety of fruits and vegetables, may originate from individual nutrients or in combinations not easily replicated by supplements.

Supplements may be added to a treatment regimen for breast, colon, prostate, and pancreatic cancer and also for the cancer weight-loss syndrome (cancer cachexia). They may also be used to counteract the effects of chemotherapy and radiation.

Supplements should be prescribed to cancer patients based on careful and continuous review of the scientific data supporting them as appropriate. Some need supplements to offset side effects, combat the metabolic syndrome, aid in the delivery of medication, and to make up for any dietary lack because of inability to eat enough. Supplements can also be used to improve insulin sensitivity in those patients with evidence of the metabolic syndrome. In addition, supplements help other health-related conditions, such as hot flashes, while patients are getting treatment.

Supplements play an adjunctive role to the far more important dietary, exercise, and stress-reduction interventions of my program. Generally, the regimen for treating early-stage cancer includes a daily multivitamin along with additional vitamin C, omega-3 fatty acids, and other nutrients.

The goals of adding supplements to treatment are to:

* Enhance and support the effectiveness of treatment
* Reduce the toxic effects of treatment
* Limit insulin resistance
* Counteract dietary inadequacy

Keep Supplements in Perspective

Unfortunately, many patients come to me to help sort out the numerous claims and promises of "natural" supplements, based on limited evidence. In addition, many distrust conventional therapies that, while toxic, are often highly effective. Some will even avoid conventional treatment in lieu of diet, supplements, and a variety of alternative, unproven therapies to treat their cancer. As Michael Lerner said in his acclaimed book on alternative treatments and cancer, *Choices in Healing*, no cancers have been consistently cured by alternative therapy. He believes strongly, as do I, that the core of integrative treatments—nutrition, physical activity, and stress reduction—work most effectively in the context of the best conventional therapy available. Some practitioners and patients resist this but the overwhelming majority of patients are seeking just this approach. By recognizing the crucial importance of the metabolic syndrome and its consequences for tumor progression and outcome, we hope to convince more doctors to explain to their patients the value of these integrative approaches.

In my second year of practice I briefly cared for Patrick, a thirty-five-year-old violinist with a national symphony orchestra. He had Hodgkin's disease and had gone from one doctor to another seeking a nonconventional approach to his disease. His resistance to conventional medicine came from a long-held belief in protecting his body—and his musical ability—from the toxicity of drugs and radiation. He was looking for something to strengthen his immune system and cure his disease. For three months, I tried to convince Patrick that he needed medical treatment; that there was a 90 percent cure rate for his disease with radiation or chemotherapy. Hoping to win him over, we spent this time negotiating, while he continued to take over thirty separate supplements prescribed by previous practitioners.

Patrick's philosophy was unshakable but, unlike other oncologists, I did not want to dismiss him. I wanted to help him with symptoms and gain his trust. I would not offer alternative treatments because I believed they would not work, and it would be unethical and dangerous.

Patrick left my practice after several months to continue his search. Meanwhile, his disease progressed with constant fevers and weight loss. A few months later, his brother called me with news of Patrick's death. They had gone to a clinic in South America that promised to cure Patrick. When they arrived, they were taken to a run-down motel in a poor section of town. Patrick's brother and a friend who had accompanied him immediately refused to allow Patrick to go into the "clinic." He died on the way home.

This early experience affected the nature of my practice as much as did my preceding years of medical and nutritional training. While valuing more in passing years the role of good nutrition and the careful and selected use of supplements, I continue to believe that conventional treatment must remain at the heart of care. On the other hand, if we fail to truly understand what our patients are seeking as partners in care, we can miss an important opportunity for healing. Our recommendations for good, integrative therapies must be made with the same rigor and thought as our prescriptions for chemotherapy or radiation. While the risks are far different, we remain obliged to follow sound medical judgment, given the uncertainties and limited evidence.

Fear of Treatment Side Effects

Most patients do understand the value of cancer treatments, though they are often frightened of their side effects. They seek help in sorting out the conflicting claims on diet and what supplements they should or shouldn't take. The common refrain heard from most is, "What can I take to build up my immune system?" They are worried that treatments might weaken their immunity, making them more vulnerable to a return of their cancer. Chemotherapy does compromise the immune system and create an increase of bacterial, viral, or even fungal infections. However, the immune system has little to do with protecting us from the progression of most cancers such as breast, colon, prostate, and pancreas. While immune therapies, including the use of monoclonal antibodies and tumor vaccines, are growing in importance in cancer care, the dream of "empowering our own immune system" to control our cancers has not borne fruit. Despite this, patients hold tenaciously to this belief and reinforce it with hundreds of dollars worth of "immune-boosting" supplements.

By carefully educating patients about the nature of cancer, the role of tumor promotion in the natural history of cancer, and the growing evidence for the role of insulin resistance in enhancing tumor growth, impairing outcomes, and potentially interfering with their therapy, we can place the role of diet and even the judicious use of supplements on firmer scientific ground.

More typical of my patients is Alice, sixty-four, who had breast cancer. She is now off active therapy but came in one day with a shopping bag full of vitamins. Many physicians would tell her, "Stop those useless vitamins," rather than educating her about the risks and potential, but unproven, benefits of supplement use. By education they could reach a truce to protect the patient from multiple, overlapping, and potentially toxic doses of some vitamins and wean her down to a simple combination of supplements based on strong evidence of benefit.

How Supplements Interact with Cancer Treatment

Nutritional supplements can sometimes interact with drugs and increase or decrease the action level of the drug. This leads to toxicity or loss of benefit from chemotherapy. Supplements may directly cause adverse side effects if they are taken in inappropriate doses or combined with other drugs, supplements, or food. When you have cancer, there is concern—though largely unproven—that some nutrient supplements may even enhance tumor growth or reduce effectiveness of medical treatment. Antioxidant components of many supplements may interfere with some chemotherapy agents or radiation. For those reasons, you must always let your doctor know about any supplements that you are taking or thinking about taking. On the other hand, appropriate supplements aid symptom relief and enhance treatment. However, they are never a substitute for good medical therapy and must be taken only with the approval of your doctor. And your doctor should always provide you with supporting literature for any recommended supplements.

I don't want you to go out and buy any of the supplements mentioned in this book until you talk it over with your physician. Every person is unique and what works for one does not necessarily work for another. The programs mentioned here are only meant to illustrate use and must be tailored for the individual. High doses of vitamins and micronutrient supplements should not be recommended during the active phase of chemotherapy, but modest doses of vitamins C, D, E, and selenium, often through a simple multivitamin, are encouraged.

Cancer and the accompanying treatments may raise the level of oxidative stress in the body. In addition, food aversions common during treatment may prevent you from getting enough antioxidants in your diet. The use of higher nutrient doses remains under investigation but there is suggestion of potential benefit in selected areas.

Supplements are always used in conjunction with diet guidelines in an overall nutrition program after the treatment has ended, and during treatment for patients who need to control other conditions, such as heart disease or menopausal symptoms. They are used to reduce the metabolic syndrome in overweight and insulin-resistant patients.

Ask your pharmacist if he or she checks supplements as well as prescribed medications in what is known as a "safe supplement program." This means they will check for interactions with drugs and other medications and supplements.

Most patients at some time take one or more nutrient supplements, often without medical guidance and frequently from uncertain sources with limited quality assurance and little consideration for risk or benefit. Because of that risk, there are some things to keep in mind.

* Always ask your doctor about the supplement before you take it.
* Buy only reputable brands from reputable manufacturers.
* Read the label thoroughly.
* Follow the guidelines for correct storage of the supplement.
* Follow the dosage guidelines on the label.
* Understand the amount you are taking and why.
* Don't increase the amount of the supplement because you believe if one pill works, then two will work better.
* Beware of advertising claims, which are almost always exaggerated, and not always based on scientific research.
* Find out if the supplement will cause interactions with drugs you are taking.
* Don't use supplements if the expiration date is past.
* If you have side effects, stop taking the supplement and call your doctor.

Vitamins and Minerals for Overall Health

Individualized programs for cancer patients may involve the addition of a single multivitamin to their daily regimen three to four days after their chemotherapy treatment. This helps if they are not eating enough during treatment and risk side effects with inadequate antioxidants and other nutrients. One single multivitamin is usually adequate but some patients also need specific vitamins.

Vitamins need to be limited to a level that won't interfere with the chemotherapy. For example, vitamins A, C, and E and folic acid should not exceed safe limits or they can interfere with treatment. (However, vegetables and fruits containing these vitamins don't interfere and they provide synergy far greater than supplements.)

Folate

Also known as folic acid, folate is an essential micronutrient involved in the regulation of genes. It is important in the metabolism of certain amino acids and in maintaining your body's chemical balance. When you don't have enough folate, it throws off the levels of other B vitamins, too. This is why folate is added to cereals, pastas, and orange juice. It is found naturally in spinach, legumes, and asparagus. (It is a critically important nutrient for pregnant women, because not getting enough can result in a low-birth-weight baby and increase the risk of neural-tube-closure defects, leading to spina bifida.) Folate also seems to blunt the increased risk of breast cancer associated with alcohol intake.

While folate is important in preventing disease, if you already have colon or breast cancer, avoid taking supplements because folate can interfere with cellular DNA and enhance the growth of malignant cells.

Selenium

Selenium is an essential trace mineral that helps support the body's natural glutathione antioxidant pathway. It is found in varying levels in plants, depending on the soil. The eastern United States, where soils are typically low in selenium, has a higher rate of many cancers than people living in the high plains of northern Nebraska and the Dakotas, where the soil has high levels of selenium.

In a skin cancer prevention trial in men in the Northeast conducted by the University of Arizona, men were given selenium or a placebo. After several years of follow-up they had no difference in the incidence of skin cancer. However, they had a marked reduction in many cancers including lung, colon, and prostate. This study is now being replicated in several large trials around the nation, including the SELECT trial, studying both selenium and vitamin E in preventing prostate cancer.

Whole grains like oatmeal and brown rice are rich in selenium, depending on where they are grown. Selenium is also found in lean meat and seafood. Brazil nuts are also a very reliable source. However, too much selenium can lead to adverse side effects, including brittle nails and bad breath. Avoid supplements of over 300 micrograms.

Vitamin E

Vitamin E has multiple forms, including the major ones: gamma tocopherol and alpha tocopherol. The latter is the form of the vitamin that circulates in the body in the highest levels and is the most potent antioxidant. Until recently, it has been the major form of vitamin E supplement. In fact, we only recently recognized that alpha tocopherol supplements will actually lower the level of gamma tocopherol in the body. Foods with vitamin E, such as certain vegetable oils and wheat germ, often contain a balanced ratio of the different forms of the vitamin. However, it may be difficult for cancer patients to get all they need from their diet, so supplements are often called for. Mixed tocopherols are the most effective supplements because they contain both gamma and alpha tocopherols in the correct ratio.

Using a mixed tocopherol is wise because there are still conflicting reports on the value of vitamin E. A recent study of 135,000 participants in nineteen different trials suggested that taking more than 400 units of vitamin E could shorten life, while taking less than 200 units seemed to reduce mortality. This study has been criticized by many researchers in the field, but it raises concerns that even standard doses of vitamins may not have the benefit we have assumed. Of concern is a recent study of patients with head and neck cancer who were given 400 IUs of vitamin E as alpha tocopherol during radiation therapy and continued for several years thereafter. These patients had an increased risk of second cancers, raising concerns about the long-term safety of higher doses of alpha tocopherol in cancer patients.

While some studies have supported a role for taking up to 400 units of vitamin E in preventing prostate cancer, a large study from the American Cancer Society has not shown any impact of the most common supplement, alpha tocopherol, in reducing prostate cancer risk. However, more evidence is showing benefit for gamma tocopherol, abundant in soy and other foods, which appears to have a potential benefit in reducing prostate cancer risk. Alpha tocopherol as well as selenium seem to play a role in preventing prostate cancer only when gamma tocopherol levels are adequate. Gamma tocopherol, while a less potent antioxidant in vitamin E, has significantly more anti-inflammatory effects. Thus a combination of alpha and gamma tocopherols is the best way to use vitamin E, with a limit of less than 100 IUs of alpha tocopherol daily.

Calcium

For most of the past three decades, the U.S. Department of Agriculture and the American Heart Association have recommended low-fat diets to help prevent heart disease. Did this concern for excess fat make people give up cheese, milk, and other healthful foods? Overall intake of milk has declined significantly over the last three decades as the prevalence of obesity and type 2 diabetes has increased. Nine of ten women, seven of ten men, and three of four teenagers don't get enough calcium. After the age of eleven no age group achieves even 75 percent of the calcium it needs. Calcium deficiency is now a public health problem. Low calcium intake is one of the most significant nutrient deficiencies identified in the federal government's Healthy People 2010 report.

Studies show that calcium decreases cancer cell proliferation and blocks the tumor effects of dietary fats. In a study published in the *New England Journal of Medicine,* a 1,200 milligram daily dose of calcium reduced the risk of colon tumors both forming and recurring.

Calcium appears to have some role in the regulation of the cells lining the colon, although it is not entirely clear how this works. Diets supplemented with calcium seem to minimize bile acids, and laboratory studies suggest that calcium can inactivate carcinogens from fatty acids because it has an emulsifying action, much the way detergent cuts the grease in a frying pan. Studies now indicate that increasing levels of calcium may reduce the transformation to colon cancer. A high-calcium diet has also been linked to reduction in insulin resistance and diabetes.

A healthy diet with low-fat dairy products accompanied by adequate calcium may be essential. Fat-free milk and yogurt are a good way to get calcium and protein. Cheese contains calcium but is also a high solid (saturated) fat food.

Older adults need calcium supplements because they rarely get enough in their diet. You would need to drink a quart of milk a day to get adequate amounts of calcium in your diet. As a result, most adults need to take supplements of calcium with vitamin D added. Vitamin D helps the body absorb calcium and is essential for bone mineralization.

Chewable calcium supplements are the best form to use because you grind it into smaller doses more easily absorbed. Calcium citrate is better than calcium carbonate because it is easier to absorb. Caltrate Plus chewable is what I recommend. Most cancer patients should take between 1,200 and 1,500 micrograms of calcium daily.

Vitamin D

We need vitamin D in order to absorb calcium. Thus, you may notice that most milk is fortified with vitamin D. But too much calcium in the diet can inhibit our body's ability to metabolize vitamin D. For example, prostate cancer patients should avoid too much calcium, but they need vitamin D. Medical scientists have recently discovered that vitamin D may thwart tumors.

About 90 percent of the vitamin D your body gets comes from sun exposure, which prompts the skin to produce a biologically inert form of the substance, which is then converted in the kidneys to an active form, a hormone called calcitriol. Calcitriol plays an important role in controlling cell growth and maturation. Colon, prostate, and breast cells carry the protein receptor that binds to calcitriol. In fact, prostate cells may even make this hormone themselves to inhibit their own growth. Male hormones are the gas pedal driving the prostate's growth, and vitamin D might be the brake. Large doses of vitamin D or the hormone calcitriol can inhibit the proliferation of cancerous cells, according to lab studies. It may also convert tumor cells into normal cells to prevent them from spreading, and even kill them. Scientists are trying to learn whether calcitriol might be a potent cancer therapy, but high doses could be toxic. This hormone prevents the growth of malignant cells. Although still controversial, some researchers are looking into vitamin D as a possible remedy and clinical trials are underway to see if the vitamin can treat tumors or bolster chemotherapy.

Blacks may get less vitamin D naturally, as their skin does not absorb as much of the sun's rays. This may partly explain why prostate cancer is twice as common in black men as in white men. Studies have shown that people in relatively sun-deprived regions or with low vitamin D levels appear at greater risk for a variety of cancers. Men in Maine are 50 percent more likely to die of prostate cancer than men in Florida, according to one study.

Based on death certificates in twenty-four states, researchers at the National Cancer Institute reported that the chances of dying from breast, colon, ovarian, and prostate cancer were reduced by about 10 to 27 percent for people in the sunniest areas, compared with those to the north.

Improving the Effectiveness of Chemotherapy

A future role for supplements may be evolving as research demonstrates the possible synergy between conventional chemotherapy and natural products.

Feverfew

There are two very provocative studies about taxanes, the drug class that includes paclitaxel (Taxol) and docetaxel (Taxotere). In one study in the journal *Oncogene,* parthenolides, a group of compounds present in the herb feverfew, a popular remedy for migraine headaches, was found to reverse tumor resistance to Taxol in cell cultures. When a woman with breast cancer did not respond to Taxol, we gave her some feverfew and gamma-linolenic acid (GLA). This reversed her resistance to the Taxol, resulting in a six-month remission and improving her quality of life. Possible side effects of feverfew include mouth ulcers, altered taste, increased heart rate, and skin rash. However, we do not recommend patients take this supplement at this time. We hope that future clinical trials will document the synergistic benefit of these compounds with chemotherapy.

Gamma-Linolenic Acid (GLA)

Gamma-linolenic acid is a polyunsaturated fatty acid found in high levels in borage and evening primrose oils. It is an omega-6 anti-inflammatory and it may improve chemotherapy activity, especially with women taking Taxol for breast cancer. In an animal study of breast cancer published in the *European Journal of Cancer,* GLA was found to significantly increase the effectiveness of the taxanes in killing cancer cells. It may reverse resistance to Taxol, according to animal studies. It has also been suggested that GLA supplements may directly inhibit breast tumor growth.

Similar research is indicating synergy between omega-3 fatty acids and Adriamycin, a mainstay of many cancer treatment combinations.

Animal studies show that some supplements increase the effectiveness of chemotherapy in killing cells. In fact, powerful antioxidant medications can be used along with chemotherapy. Chinese ginseng can lower cortisol levels in diabetics and improve chemotherapy but can interfere with blood clotting, so it must be used with caution.

Reducing the Toxic Effects of Treatment

As useful as chemotherapy can be for fighting cancer, it, of course, also has some toxic effects in the body. Some antioxidant compounds may reduce toxic effects to the kidneys and heart of chemotherapy drugs such as cisplatin and Adriamycin (doxorubicin).

Cardiac Effects

The natural compound coenzyme Q_{10} may have similar cardioprotective benefits to the drug Zinocard when used in combination with high doses of Adriamycin. Coenzyme Q_{10} is like a vitamin and provides energy and regulates metabolism and cholesterol. It is beneficial in a variety of cancers, including advanced cancer.

Prolonged use of Adriamycin can be harmful to normal heart function, so Q_{10} combined with the drug dexrazone can reduce the effect. However, additional antioxidants are necessary for patients with heart disease and those who don't get enough antioxidants in their diet. Coenzyme Q_{10}, vitamins A and E, selenium, and grapeseed extract all may help reduce the cardiac effects of cancer treatment.

Neuropathy

Chemotherapy with taxanes, cisplatins, and other drugs used in blood cancers can cause neuropathy, resulting in a numbness and tingling in the hands and feet. Alpha-lipoic acid in intravenous form will combat this. I also recommend taking vitamin B_6 twice a day along with folic acid, magnesium, and evening primrose oils. A capsaicin salve can be applied to the skin over the neuropathy to help reduce it. Antidepressant and antiseizure drugs are also effective in some cases.

Scarring from Radiation

Radiation treatment causes scar tissue to form. For example, if you had radiation to your breast, then the tissue that was the target of this repeated dose of radiation dies. It no longer functions like normal tissue. It does not absorb medications or body chemicals. It feels like a hard lump. High doses of vitamin E in combination with pentoxyfiline, a medication that alters cytokine production in tissues, may limit the scarring caused by radiation therapy, including the skin and possibly fibrosis of the lung. This should be used only in a trial setting with a doctor's guidance and for short periods because of the uncertain risks associated with long-term use of vitamin E.

Combating Insulin Resistance

Some nutritional supplements are used to complement diet and exercise to improve insulin function without interfering with your cancer therapy. These include lower doses of vitamin C, mixed tocopherols (a balanced mixture of vitamin E compounds), alpha-lipoic acid, omega-3 fatty acids, and calcium as well as micronutrients such as magnesium. We give magnesium to patients with insulin resistance only if they cannot get enough in their diet. This helps control high blood pressure. Magnesium is found in almost every type of food but the highest amounts are in sea salt, kelp, wheat germ, blackstrap molasses, and oats and nuts.

Treating Cancer Cachexia

Cancer cachexia is a wasting condition caused by certain cancers (see chapter 3) even when there is adequate nourishment. It reflects a complex metabolic change spurred by increasing levels of cytokines that cause progressive loss in muscle mass.

Often, abnormal glucose metabolism with insulin resistance accompanies this state. While the only effective therapy is ultimately the control of the underlying cancer, certain supplements may play a therapeutic role. High doses of omega-3 supplements have been shown to improve the weight and overall nutritional status as well as accompanying immune dysfunction present in some patients with this syndrome. A recently identified protein compound, proteolysis-inducing factor (PIF), has been identified as being partly responsible for the muscle loss. The action of the supplements may suppress this PIF protein.

Patients with this condition should take omega-3 fatty acids with meals to prevent muscle breakdown. Anti-inflammatory medications such as ibuprofen may enhance the effect of fatty acids in reducing inflammation and improving nutritional status. Megace is a medication that improves appetite and increases weight gain. I also want these patients to take one can of a nutritional supplement such as ProSure two to three times a day. Multivitamin and antioxidant supplements reduce oxidative stress and improve wound healing.

Exercise will help rebuild muscle mass and improve aerobic conditioning, which is essential to reduce weight loss, fatigue, and emotional distress.

Combating Oxidative Stress and Inflammation

Cancer treatment by its very nature wreaks havoc in the body and leads to oxidative stress and inflammation. By killing all the cancer cells, the drugs are also killing healthy cells that have a job to do. This leads to oxidative stress.

When you see rust on iron, or the flesh of an apple turning brown, this is oxidative stress at work. Your body is constantly reacting to oxygen as part of the production of energy. Unstable molecules inside the body known as free radicals are unleashed by this process. These molecules are products of the normal cellular process. They are seeking mates so they can become stable by interacting with the nearest molecule. It is the job of antioxidants to mop up these free radicals and neutralize them.

The metabolic processes that produce antioxidants in your body are controlled and influenced by your genetic makeup as well as by diet, smoking, and pollution to which you are exposed. When we have less quality in our diet, we are exposed to more free radicals than ever. By increasing antioxidants in our diet, we defend ourselves better against oxidative stress.

The body has some of its own antioxidants, such as alpha-lipoic acid (ALA), which increases the effectiveness of vitamins C and E and some other antioxidants. Ask your doctor about N-acetylcysteine (NAC), a potent antioxidant that inhibits the carcinogens in tobacco smoke and helps maintain healthy lung function. It can lower cholesterol levels by up to 70 percent and inhibits the oxidation of LDL, the bad cholesterol.

Food-based antioxidants include vitamins E, C, and beta-carotene, the precursor of vitamin A. Trace elements that are components of antioxidant enzymes include selenium, copper, zinc, and manganese. While it's best to get these antioxidants in your food, the use of a daily multivitamin with these vitamins and minerals will help combat oxidative stress.

A chronic inflammatory state also fosters proliferation of abnormal cells and stimulates cancer cells by increasing angiogenesis, the process of new blood vessels growing to feed cancer cells.

Omega-3 fats have an important anti-inflammatory effect. They reduce prostaglandins involved in the inflammatory response. (Refer back to chapter 7 for more about omega-3 and omega-6 fatty acids.) The role of these agents as well as natural products such as omega-3 fatty acids is growing beyond the initial role in treating pain and local inflammation. They also prevent weight loss in patients with cancer cachexia.

If you don't get enough omega-3 fatty acids in your diet—and many people, especially cancer patients, do not—then you need supplements. Omega-3 influences the inflammatory state, improves insulin resistance, alters the synthesis of prostaglandins, and decreases cell growth.

These omega-3 supplements should be taken three times a day with meals. But begin by taking them only once a day for a few days so that your digestive system gets used to them. They can cause bloating. The dose is about 1 gram. Some supplements are less fishy-tasting, so read the labels and do some research first. Ask your doctor about them.

✳ **Fish oil supplements.** Fish oil with omega-3 improves appetite and helps avoid loss of lean body mass. Too much, however, can cause belching and diarrhea. Avoid preparations that also contain vitamins A and D. Many doctors advise patients not to take these supplements because they may cause bleeding. However, this won't happen if you use 3 grams or less a day. Although fish oil supplements can provide a hefty dose of omega-3s, they raise serious concerns for some people. Diabetics should note that fish oil supplements can affect blood sugar control. People with bleeding disorders and people taking blood-thinning medications such as aspirin should not use fish oil supplements because they decrease the ability of the blood to clot.

✳ **Docosahexanoic acid (DHA).** Known simply as DHA for obvious reasons of pronunciation, docosahexanoic acid is an omega-3 fatty acid supplement.

✳ **Flaxseed.** Flaxseed (alpha-linoleic acid) is the best omega-3 supplement. It's a very important antioxidant and regenerates cells and improves glucose control. It will cause more bowel movements, however. Use one tablespoon of bruised seeds two to three times a day and drink lots of water. Sprinkle some seeds on your oatmeal in the morning so your cereal will contain good soluble fiber as well as omega-3.

✳ **Gamma-linolenic acid (GLA).** This comes from evening primrose oil, borage oil, and black currant plants. It is also found in human breast milk. GLA combats inflammation and improves the effectiveness of Taxol and Taxotere. It has been suggested that GLA supplements may inhibit the growth of cancer cells and reduce tumor invasion. Lab studies have shown that GLA can inhibit the growth of some cancer cells, but there's no evidence yet that it can prevent or treat cancer. Human studies are being done to evaluate the role of essential fatty acids on the growth of cancer cells.

GLA supplements are available in liquid and capsules. GLA also works with omega-3 fatty acids in limiting inflammation. We frequently combine GLA with fish oil in patients with significant evidence of C-RP and other signs of systemic inflammation.

Antioxidants and Anti-inflammatory Supplements

Here is a list of other antioxidants and anti-inflammatory supplements that are often used in our program with cancer therapy. Again, don't use these without the advice or your doctor.

* Salicin (Salix alba willow bark extract) is often called "herbal aspirin" and has been used in Chinese medicine for centuries to relieve pain and lower fever. The salicylic acid in white willow bark lowers the body's levels of prostaglandins, which cause inflammation. It takes longer to begin acting than aspirin, but its effects may last longer. Unlike aspirin, it doesn't irritate the stomach. However, there is a risk involved for those allergic to aspirin.

* Boswellia (boswellic acid) inhibits the inflammatory response. It is also known as boswellin or "Indian frankincense" and comes from a tree that grows in the dry hills of India. Indian healers have used the anti-inflammatory properties of the tree's gummy resin. Unlike conventional nonsteroidal anti-inflammatory drugs (NSAIDs) such as ibuprofen, it does not irritate the stomach.

* Ginger has long been used in cooking and medicine. It is used to combat nausea and is also an anti-inflammatory. The stem of the plant contains gingerols, which give the plant its color and flavor.

* Turmeric, a common ingredient in curry powder, is an important antioxidant and anti-inflammatory. It is a spice widely used in Indian cooking. The active ingredient is curcumin, which has antioxidant and anti-inflammatory properties.

* Bromelain is the name of a group of powerful protein-digesting enzymes found in the pineapple plant that reduce muscle and tissue inflammation. It is a natural blood thinner and anti-inflammatory. It is generally safe, even in high doses, but people with ports for chemotherapy must be careful because it may cause them to bleed.

* Milk thistle (Silybum marianum) is a digestive tonic that can reduce inflammation. It stimulates regeneration of liver tissue and protects it from toxic substances such as alcohol and certain drugs. It may also intensify the effects of drugs that decrease blood sugar levels (hypoglycemic drugs).

* Green tea is a great source of polyphenols and antioxidants known as catechins in higher concentrations than black tea. Another ingredient, circumen, reduces inflammation. Green tea also reduces DNA damage and angiogenesis, the growth of blood vessels that supply the cancer cells. It has less caffeine than black tea, which is fermented. The average amount of caffeine in an eight-ounce cup of green tea is twenty-five to fifty grams, compared to forty to sixty grams for black tea. (Coffee has 100 to 120.) Green tea comes from leaves that are immediately steamed (unfermented) prior to drying. Black tea comes from leaves that are crushed and exposed to the air for several hours (fully fermented or oxidized). Black tea is a less effective antioxidant, but is sometimes used to treat diarrhea. I recommend three cups a day of green tea as an antioxidant and as a way to get fluids.

Traditional Chinese Herbal Remedies

In some therapy programs we include the careful use of Chinese herbal teas. Herbal medicines are always used with great caution during active chemotherapy, with awareness of potential drug-herb interactions. Further, many herbs are avoided because of their known risks and side effects. If you have breast cancer, avoid red clover because it can stimulate breast cancer cells. Also use caution with any of the phytoestrogen compounds, including soy and dong quai.

Beijing University and Memorial Sloan-Kettering Cancer Center are collaborating in studies of the effects of Chinese herbal medicine to aid in nutrition, improve immune function, and reduce fatigue. My own practice is currently embarked on a study of the effectiveness of traditional Chinese herbal remedies in treating the postchemotherapy fatigue syndrome, particularly common after breast cancer. This fatigue often comes with mild depression or anxiety and an increase in circulating cytokines that reflect low-level inflammation.

There are many forms of traditional Chinese medicine. Techniques and procedures that the Chinese healers have been using for centuries include acupuncture, acupressure, Chinese massage (see chapter 13) qigong, and tai chi (see chapter 12). A Chinese physician with both an MD and extensive training in China in traditional Chinese medicine runs the program used in my practice. By understanding conventional medical practice as well as the physical nature of illness, this physician appreciates the benefits and limitations of acupuncture.

Supplements to Avoid

Some supplements should never be used. Soy, lycopene, and some flavonoids contain many healthful phytonutrients and are effective in their natural food state, but as supplements, in high doses they can be risky.

* Soy isoflavones highly concentrated in supplements are potentially dangerous for breast cancer patients. Most isoflavones are weak estrogens, but some soy actually causes breast cells to proliferate. Genistein, an isoflavone in soy, may actually interfere with tamoxifen treatment. Soy-based foods such as tofu are okay.

* Lycopene is a nutrient found in tomatoes and watermelon, among other vegetables and fruits. Lack of this nutrient has been found to be one of the strongest factors in the risk of prostate cancer. As a result, lycopene supplements have been suggested for use in lowering PSA levels in men with prostate cancer. On rare occasions I give 10 to 20 milligrams a day to prostate cancer patients who cannot get enough of this nutrient in their diet and when there are no other options. However, we have no long-term evidence that the supplements act as well as the actual food and they can be toxic. Therefore, they should be used only with care, under a doctor's guidance.

* Red clover is a phytoestrogen and can stimulate breast cancer cells.

* Mixed carotenoids and flavonoids are powerful antioxidants found in a variety of vegetables and fruits. And you should try to eat them that way. As extracts, they are often used inappropriately and can be either toxic or ineffective. Mixed carotenoids (natural carotene extracts) include alpha-carotene, beta-carotene, lutein, lycopene, and xanthins. Natural carotenoids are found in fruits and vegetables that are yellow, orange, or red. Generally, the darker the color, the more concentrated the carotenoid. Some are also converted into vitamin A. Mixed flavonoids are a complex group of

chemicals (cirsiliol, quercetin, rutin, hesperetin, hesperi-din, kaempferol) with different but often overlapping func-tions. They are antioxidants that help the body delay or slow down oxidative damage to cells and tissue. Natural flavonoids are found in apples, onions, and some beverages such as tea, coffee, beer, wine, and fruit drinks. Foods con-taining beta-carotenes were associated with reduction in lung cancer incidence. However, in a cancer prevention study in Scandinavia, male smokers were given supplements of beta-carotene or vitamin E or both to reduce lung cancer risk. Those patients taking the supplements had increased lung cancer. This was replicated in a study of beta-carotene in smokers exposed to asbestos. These studies are reminders of the unpredictable risk when taking seemingly safe sup-plements in high doses and the important role that food, rather than vitamin supplements, plays in true cancer pre-vention.

✳   Resveratrol is a flavonoid found in red wine (see chapter 6), mulberries, and eucalyptus. It is in some grapes but not in grape juice. It is an anti-inflammatory and aids in the effec-tiveness of chemotherapy. It's also a weak phytoestrogen and antioxidant. Resveratrol in red wine helps reduce the risk of heart attack and also raises good cholesterol levels. However, supplements with resveratrol are not regulated, may contain fillers, and should be avoided.

Supplemental Medications

Some over-the-counter remedies, like aspirin, and prescription drugs, like the statins—drugs used to lower cholesterol levels—may aid in cancer treatment as well because of their powerful anti-inflammatory effect. Preliminary data even suggest that statins may reduce risk of some cancers, including breast and colon. The statins are not toxic except for rare cases of muscle or liver damage, which is usually reversible when you stop the drug.

Aspirin and other anti-inflammatory drugs (NSAIDs) are also said to reduce deaths from colon cancer, but only in the earliest stages, according to current research. It is believed to stop the growth of polyps in the colon that might become aggressive over time. It might be aspirin's ability to block production of prostaglandins. Many studies show that regular aspirin users have less colon cancer.

The anti-inflammatory drugs known as COX-2 inhibitors, used for arthritis pain, also inhibit prostaglandins. Like aspirin, the COX-2 inhibitor has a role in colon cancer prevention and treatments for a variety of cancers, including those of the lung, pancreas, and breast. However, because of the growing evidence that this group of drugs may actually increase heart attack risk, attention is returning to nonspecific anti-inflammatory drugs such as aspirin and other nonsteroidals, including ibuprofen. Despite this new information on risk, recent trials are confirming a benefit to celecoxib (Celebrex) in reducing the risk of colon cancer development in patients with genetic risk factors such as familial polyposis. This has created great concern among oncologists, who have increasingly viewed these COX-2 inhibitors as exciting agents because of their anti-inflammatory and anti-angiogenesis effects. The balance will be decided only by future studies and careful weighing of pros and cons.

Use over-the-counter drugs with caution. As mentioned, your doctor should know what you are taking, especially because it may interfere with your treatment. Even after treatment, be sure to know how such drugs affect your health. People take so many over-the-counter medications in this country that the National Consumer's League joined by the U.S. Food and Drug Administration launched a campaign in 2004 aimed at educating the public about taking precautions. Misuse of pain relievers and NSAIDs increases intestinal bleeding and can cause other serious side effects, such as damage to the liver. If you have questions about over-the-counter medications, check the National Consumers League Web site at www. nclnet.org and look for the Take with Care program.

Supplements for Specific Cancers

Nutritional interventions should be designed for each cancer patient individually, but there are some cancers that generally require more specific supplements. In addition to a multivitamin and antioxidants and anti-inflammatories, some patients need additional supplements. I encourage taking multivitamins with your largest meal of the day because oxidative stress often rises after eating, particularly with high-fat meals.

Colon Cancer

For colon cancer, I recommend calcium supplements of 1,200 to 1,500 milligrams a day, as well as consuming as much milk and other low-fat dairy products as possible. Cultured nonfat yogurt is a good way to increase dairy and it is easy to digest. Fish high in omega-3 fatty acids should be eaten as often as possible. Folate should be limited, but take 200 micrograms of selenium supplements. I also recommend an aspirin a day, unless you are on active chemotherapy or are at risk of increased bleeding. Always check with your doctor first.

Breast Cancer

A supplemental vitamin E of mixed tocopherols with 100 IUs or less of alpha tocopherol should be taken by breast cancer patients, along with flaxseed and soy foods such as tofu. You may need additional folate, but check with your physician about dosage. However, avoid taking isoflavone supplements, which interfere with tamoxifen. Concentrated soy products are also dangerous. Alcohol should be limited.

Prostate Cancer

Men with prostate cancer should restrict fat to 20 percent of calories. Men are also encouraged to increase soy intake. Eat cooked tomatoes (for the lycopene) once or twice every day. With this cancer, too much calcium is not good because it turns off vitamin D, which is crucial. But do consume low-fat milk or other dairy products three times a day to limit insulin resistance. Remember, it's the protein in the milk that's important here. Add sources of selenium, folate, and vitamin E to your diet.

NOW YOU see how complex the body's natural biochemical system is. This is why you can do more harm than good with do-it-yourself remedies. Always consult your doctor before taking supplements. If he or she does not think they are necessary, or puts them all down as ineffective, then seek out more medical advice.

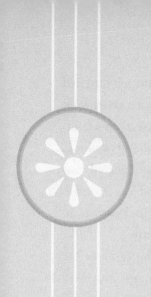

CHAPTER 10

Beat the Fatigue of Cancer Treatment and Lower Insulin Resistance with Exercise

EXERCISE, EXERCISE, EXERCISE! This is the only way to combat cancer treatment fatigue and it often works. It not only improves your energy and mood, it shortens periods of low blood counts. Nobody expects you to participate in a triathlon while you are undergoing cancer treatment. You may feel weak and tired much of the time. But there are ways of walking—and breathing—that will help you feel surprisingly energetic.

There is mounting evidence that physical activity protects us against cancer over and above its proven ability to prevent weight gain. Being physically active resets several of the body's functions in precisely the same way that obesity and being overweight disrupt them. It's already been proven that people who are active at work or at play have less risk of colon and breast cancer, and the evidence is growing that it helps other cancers as well.

Physical activity also aids in cancer treatment. Anne felt fatigued from her chemotherapy, and I advised her to go out for a short walk every day. I told her to pick a place that is serene and walk at a comfortable pace for thirty minutes. Along with the action of walking, she was breathing deeply and relieving stress. Anne reported that the daily walk had indeed made her feel less tired and less stressful. And of course, that activity was keeping her insulin levels down, so her chemotherapy treatment could be the most effective.

Louise, fifty-seven, is another good example. She came to me eight years ago with early-stage breast cancer. Her tumor was small and estrogen sensitive and she was treated with a lumpectomy and follow-up radiation. She did not need chemotherapy and refused tamoxifen. At the time of diagnosis, she was more than forty pounds overweight and a couch potato, doing virtually no physical activity. We urged Louise to set a goal to lose twenty pounds over six to twelve months through diet and increasing exercise. Despite the recommendations, along with several follow-up meetings explaining the implications of her weight, she continued with her poor eating habits and limited activity. We didn't see Louise for five years, but when she returned, she had gained another fifteen pounds and now had endometrial cancer. She also had poorly controlled hypertension and diabetes, which made her a poor candidate for surgery. Radiation therapy was now her only treatment option. This case illustrates the potential danger of weight gain and failure to exercise.

It's Never Too Late to Begin

Even if you have been sedentary all your life, you can begin exercise now and still gain protection. Moderate but frequent activity may be nearly as effective in reducing weight along with risk of cancer and cardiovascular disease when it's part of a program of weight loss and stress reduction.

Postmenopausal women who engaged in regular strenuous activity had an 18 percent lower risk of breast cancer compared to inactive women in one study. Even less strenuous physical activity, the equivalent of one and a quarter to two and a half hours a week of brisk walking, can protect you from breast cancer (not to mention heart attack and stroke).

Here are some findings:

* Women over fifty with consistently high activity had 67 percent less risk of breast cancer. The same benefit was not noted for women under fifty.

* Finnish physical education teachers had a 17 percent lower risk of breast cancer than did less active language teachers.

* Women who do vigorous activity seven or more hours a week had an 18 percent reduction in risk of invasive breast cancer.

* In a German study of thirty-three women with breast cancer who received high-dose chemotherapy followed by stem cell transplantation, those who spent thirty minutes a day riding a stationary bike during their hospitalization had less diarrhea and other side effects from the chemotherapy than women who did not train. They had improved outcomes, and their body's ability to function was protected.

* A study in Canada looked at 123 women with stage 1 and 2 breast cancer. Some of the women were in a supervised exercise group and others were in a self-directed group. Women in the supervised group fared better.

* A study of seventy-two women with breast cancer in a home-based program of moderate exercise found that fatigue declined with low to moderate exercise. As the exercise level increased in duration, the level of fatigue declined.

* The American Cancer Society found that women with breast cancer who were anxious at the beginning of treatment felt less anxious after doing regular exercise.

❋ As early as the 1960s, researchers found that the risk of colon cancer increased in sedentary men. (Surprisingly, rectal cancer has not been found to share the same protection with physical activity.)

Not a Choice, But a Necessity

Theresa, thirty-seven, is a homemaker diagnosed with an aggressive breast cancer. At the time of diagnosis she had two positive lymph nodes and a hormone-negative cancer. She began a regimen of dose-dense chemotherapy with Adriamycin, cyclophosphamide and Taxol. After the first treatment, Theresa had such prolonged nausea that she needed two days in the hospital because she could not eat or drink. Once the dehydration and nausea cleared, she was reluctant to do anything physical. Before her second round of treatment, and in addition to a nutrition assessment, I had a long talk with Theresa and her husband about the importance of physical activity. After that second round of treatment Theresa began to go for a daily walk with her husband. She found it remarkable that she had fewer symptoms than with her first round of chemotherapy. She also had more rapid recovery of her blood counts, and her mood and well-being improved. Naturally, her recovery cannot be completely attributed to exercise, but her case demonstrates the importance of integrating good medical treatment with nutrition and exercise. You don't really need to rest during cancer treatment except when there are significant side effects. Exercise contributes in a big way to your sense of well-being and tolerance for treatment.

Cancer-related fatigue is partly an effect of mood and psychological stress. One of the benefits of regular exercise is the improvement in mood. Few studies have addressed the effect of exercise on tumor recurrence and mortality, but it is well known that increased weight puts you at more risk of recurrence. Increased body weight, abdominal obesity, and insulin resistance aid in cancer progression. This effect is blunted by regular exercise.

How Exercise Affects Your Hormonal Balance

If you are overweight or inactive, you produce higher levels of hormones that spur cell division. Since cancer is a malfunction of cells during the division, this kind of rapid cell division provides greater opportunity for initiation of the disease.

* Exercise *decreases* the overproduction of sex hormones related to risk of several cancers, including breast, prostate, endometrial, and ovarian.
* Exercise increases the protein that binds to these sex hormones (testosterone as well as estrogen), thereby keeping the hormones out of circulation.
* Physical activity reduces fat deposits, which makes it harder for dietary carcinogens to be stored long term in the body.
* Physical activity improves the body's antioxidant defense systems and strengthens other immune defenses as well.
* Increasing activity has a powerful anti-inflammatory effect.
* Exercise enhances blood glucose movement into muscle and other tissue and reduces circulating insulin levels.

This last effect is shown in a study from the Pritikin Center and the University of California at Los Angeles. A group of postmenopausal women on a two-week high-fiber, low-fat diet took a daily brisk walk for forty-five to sixty minutes. They had a significant reduction in weight, body mass index, blood fats (cholesterol and triglycerides), glucose, and insulin levels as well as a C-reactive protein. This short intervention also had a significant impact on risk factors for cardiovascular disease and cancer mortality.

Getting Rid of the Abdominal Fat

Production of cortisol, the stress hormone, contributes to visceral abdominal fat. Getting rid of abdominal fat is important, but not any more difficult than losing other fat. This usually drops away as you exercise and lose weight all over. STRIDE, a program at Duke University for sedentary, overweight men and women with abnormal lipid profiles, compared varying levels of exercise, with no change in normal diet. They found a clear relationship between the intensity and duration of activity and the amount of body weight and fat lost over this period, but all three groups lost weight and body fat—including abdominal fat, waist size, and hip circumference. The most intense exercisers lost a greater amount. Even those doing less intense exercise lost weight, although not as much. However, even a small increase in activity level led to weight loss. In contrast, a control group, followed over time with no intervention, gained weight.

A minimal amount of activity is needed for weight control if there is no change in diet. Most people can achieve this with a brisk half-hour walk or a more vigorous jog for twenty minutes. At a minimum, walk six miles a week.

Learning to Be Active

According to the 2000 National Health Interview Survey, 72 percent of women and 64 percent of men get no regular exercise. Most sedentary people simply never got into the habit of activity. They don't walk. They sit behind a desk or in a car. Once you are used to that, any physical activity feels like torture.

Having cancer changes your outlook and many patients use this as a wake-up call to get rid of bad habits and form good ones—including becoming physically active.

One of the best ways to make daily exercise a habit is to find activities you enjoy and people who enjoy them with you. Valerie, fifty-five, is a suburban woman who gets up at six every morning and walks two miles around her suburb. She is joined by others at various points along the route. The women do this despite having no sidewalks.

Phyllis, sixty, lost twenty-five pounds when she joined a seniors' basketball team with her friends. She had dieted before, but admitted that she wanted to look good on the court. And of course, the exercise kept the weight off. Her team is also in the senior Olympics and having the time of their lives. Several other women on the team are cancer survivors.

In order to keep insulin levels down, you must do a minimum of thirty minutes of moderate to vigorous activity five days a week. What qualifies as vigorous activity: brisk walking, jogging, and swimming. You've likely heard this recommendation as a way to prevent cardiovascular disease and keep muscles and bones healthy. We now know you need this kind of activity to keep cancer under control, too, and to speed your recovery. A brisk walk, even heavy housework or yard work, is suitable. The key is to get moving and keep moving.

Even with fatigue and muscle and joint pain, you can incorporate exercise around your chemotherapy regimen. You can participate in low-level exercise three to four times a week for thirty or forty minutes.

By combining a graded exercise program with sound nutrition, you can avoid this weight gain, a common occurrence with chemotherapy. Don't wait until the weight gain has occurred and you are ten to thirty pounds above your pretreatment weight. Most of my patients embrace these lifestyle changes, even in the midst of treatment, because they know the payoff is a better quality of life and increased long-term survival.

Once my patients leave, I give them a conditioning program for continued wellness and prevention of cancer.

Begin a Graded Exercise Program

Talk with your doctor about an exercise program that includes both aerobic conditioning and muscle strengthening so you will feel better during chemotherapy and radiation therapy. Begin a graded exercise program of aerobics and strength or resistance training. Two or three days a week for fifteen minutes at a time begin with low-intensity aerobics—just a short walk will do. Here's a way to get started.

First, take your pulse by gently placing your finger on the side of your wrist near your thumb. Time the heartbeats for one minute. Normal resting heart rate for a fifty-year-old would be between sixty and one hundred beats a minute, with the average around seventy. The more fit you are, the lower that rate will be. The object of the aerobic exercise is to gradually get your heart rate up to one hundred while doing the exercise.

Twice a week, go for a walk that is long enough to get your heart rate up to one hundred.

Once a week, on a day you are not doing aerobic training, do some muscle strengthening with resistance bands or light dumbbells for fifteen minutes. These exercises will begin to tone your muscles.

After two weeks, increase the aerobic exercise to three times a week and the muscle strengthening to twice a week on alternate days. Build up to thirty minutes of muscle strengthening. After two months, do the aerobics four days a week.

Always drink plenty of fluids when you are exercising.

The BreathWalk

Unless your chemotherapy is mild, it would be difficult to do the BreathWalk during treatment. But it's vitally important to begin such a program after treatment to get into good physical shape and stay that way. BreathWalk, developed by Gurucharan Singh Khalsa, PhD, yogi, psychotherapist, teacher, and writer, and Yogi Bhajan, PhD, a master of kundalini and tantric yoga, combines the conscious synchronization of breathing pattern with walking steps. It is a walking-meditation program and is outlined in their book, *BreathWalk: Breathing Your Way to a Revitalized Body, Mind, and Spirit*, published by Broadway Books in 2000. Done consciously together, breathing and walking enhance your physical, emotional, and spiritual fitness. BreathWalk also alleviates exhaustion and anxiety, and helps your body and mind heal. Health improves through oxygenation to the body. Done properly, it opens the senses and quiets the mind. It can change your mood quickly. BreathWalk can be done anywhere: in the park, a mall, airport, even on your home treadmill. There is no special equipment needed.

Conscious breathing has long been an effective technique in meditation practiced by many cultures and healing traditions. Mindful meditation techniques often utilize awareness of breathing. With practice, combining the rhythmic cadence of walking with the conscious pattern of breathing provides a profound experience, capable of generating the relaxation response described first by Herbert Benson, MD, as central to the physiologic benefits of most meditative techniques. In addition, it simultaneously provides the well-described metabolic benefits of brisk walking. Remember Anne's daily walk and how it helped her treatment? It keeps your weight down and insulin resistance at bay and it lowers stress.

Conscious breathing and walking force you to be centered. It's best to learn this with a group, but you can do it alone. First, do three to five minutes of deep breathing in place to align your body and warm it up. Fill your belly rather than your chest with air. In the book, the breathing technique sounds more complicated than it really has to be. You should breathe in and out in sync with your walking. In other words, as you breathe in take four steps and as you breathe out take four steps slowly. This takes some time to measure and regulate. Use numbers or words to say silently or aloud in counting your steps.

Mary, thirty-three, a mother of four young children, was treated for leukemia. She felt like a totally new person after doing the BreathWalk and had the energy to deal with four children. Her disease made her bones ache and her treatment included medication that attacked the malfunction of the chromosome that caused her disease but made her very tired. Mary, formerly a massage therapist, was amenable to integrative treatment and she decided to join a group of my patients who were doing the BreathWalk in the community center across the street from my office.

In the first walk, Mary felt pain, lightheaded, and a bit tingly. However, it passed as she worked through it. She was afraid she couldn't do it but decided to push herself through the thirty-five-minute walk. The group walked very slowly, then rested, had lunch, and got ready for the second walk, which would last forty-five minutes.

Mary's second walk was exhilarating despite beginning it when she was extremely tired. She told me she felt so at peace after the walk, like her old self. Another advantage is that the BreathWalk makes you more aware of everything around you. Mary noticed the bark on the trees, the colors of the leaves of trees where the clouds shadowed them. She said it was like removing the goggles.

Some of my patients walk in or around the community center, but you can do BreathWalk anywhere, even on a treadmill. The important thing is to think about walking, which is something few Americans do anymore.

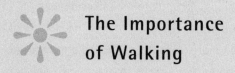

The Importance of Walking

The American environment for decades has encouraged our sedentary lifestyle. It discourages getting out of the car and off the couch. Adults won't walk three blocks to the store, and children won't walk to nearby schools. As a result, suburban people weigh six pounds more than people who live in cities and do more walking. Many people join exercise clubs that they never visit, and buy expensive home exercise machines that often go unused. Then, when they drive to the mall, they circle the parking lot searching for the spot closest to the entrance to limit their inconvenience, missing an obvious and cost-free opportunity for activity. Paradoxically, I have *never* seen anyone fighting for the most distant spot in the lot in order to combine a good walk with an errand or shopping chore.

If you try to exercise in the suburbs, you risk being hit by a car due to the dearth of sidewalks. In Europe, where cities are engineered to encourage physical activity, the accident rate is lower. The Europeans studied weigh less and live longer, too. Those in suburbs have higher blood pressure and obesity compared to city dwellers.

Another interesting study found that people who live in older homes are more likely to walk than those in newer ones. The National Cancer Institute reported that people living in homes built before 1974 are 50 percent more likely to walk a mile or more at least twenty times a month, meaning they are getting more healthy exercise than their car-bound counterparts. That's because older houses are more likely to be located in communities with sidewalks, a tight network of streets, and a business district within walking distance of residences.

No matter where you walk, the point is you need to walk every day. Until you gain more strength, try walking around the block or even in your home. Take steps in place until you are stronger. Your body needs to keep moving for it to function well.

Strength Training

If you are feeling weak from cancer treatment, you may think strength training is too tough a call for you. And besides, isn't it just for bodybuilders? Resistance training, or strength training, using weights, resistance bands (stretch bands), or training machines for muscle strengthening, has important metabolic benefits. It improves insulin sensitivity that lasts well beyond the period of exercise and it reduces your risk of muscle loss. You can do these simple repetitive exercises with small weights or low-resistance bands at first while you are sitting in a chair, or even in bed.

Start by using small dumbbells (three to five pounds) for repetitive arm exercises and leg lifts. Begin with a few repetitions (reps) and gradually work up to longer routines with heavier weights. Gradual buildup will strengthen your muscles while avoiding injury or trauma. If you use resistance bands, choose the one most easily stretched. (They come with light or difficult resistance.) They are useful for developing upper-body strength. By gripping the handles at each end, your muscles get a workout when you stretch the band between both hands, or between one foot and one hand. Most sporting goods stores carry these and they come with directions for use. Work through the exercises if you feel weak. Do ten reps once or twice a day and gradually work up to longer sessions where you do about twenty-five reps. The ideal is to do five sessions of twenty-five reps.

There are several good books and videos on strength training, so find one with basic instructions. The simplest exercise is holding the weight in your hand and raising your arm up over your head. You can do this with one arm at a time. When you gain more strength, you can do both arms at once.

Another way to build arm muscle is to do push-ups against a wall. Stand a foot or more back from a wall. Place your hands flat on the wall and lean in slowly, then push yourself back. You can build up to more reps, but there's no reason to gain speed. This exercise is good for your bones, too.

Do these exercises during quiet times at work or home. But don't think of this as a race. Think of it as a slow creation of a new habit or lifestyle.

Noreen, forty-eight, was significantly overweight with a BMI of 32 when she was diagnosed with a swollen lymph node in her right groin. She had a large ovarian mass. Her uterus and ovaries were surgically removed, but scattered small residual nodules were not removable. A CT scan showed no other visible cancer involvement, but a blood test indicated there was more cancer in her body.

At this point, Noreen came to me because she was reluctant to submit to chemotherapy for fear it would impair her immune system. Finally, after much explanation from me, she agreed to undergo six cycles of chemotherapy with Taxol and carboplatin. Afterward, there was no sign of any disease and her tumor markers returned to normal. We suggested a maintenance treatment with Taxol for a year to assure her long-term survival but she declined. However, she did agree to an aggressive nutrition and exercise program. Now her weight is down, she continues her aerobic and strength training, and is free of any signs of disease. Noreen is optimistic about her future.

Tai Chi

Tai chi is especially useful following chemotherapy to promote and restore health. It can increase flexibility and reduce stress. It improves balance and coordination, especially in older people. Tai chi is particularly useful for people recovering from chemotherapy-induced fatigue. It is not the same as strength training in that it doesn't make your muscles stronger. The slow, graceful movements increase flexibility and improve balance and circulation. The goal is to return the body and mind to its original pure and healthy state. It has been described as a form of meditation in motion where the continuity of its movements, combined with the devotion of one's undivided attention, heal and revitalize both the body and mind.

The physical component of tai chi consists of movements aimed at achieving balance, such as correcting angles, squaring hips, controlling the step and the transfer of weight, turning constantly in spirals, opening and closing, centering the trunk, and stretching and relaxing the spine. The movements are gentle, continuous, and circular.

Many find the massagelike movements of tai chi to be effective therapy for a wide range of health problems. The extra degree of stretching and turning in each movement improves health. With practice, these movements affect all body systems. Tai chi can reduce body fat, raising the possibility that it may prevent heart disease. It is one of the few exercises that is appropriate for anybody, regardless of condition. It can even be done in a bed or chair. Tai chi is particularly useful for the frail elderly because it improves balance and flexibility, thus reducing the risk of falls and subsequent fractures common in this age group. It may also help retard bone loss typical in older, inactive people.

Tai chi helped Pauline, who was overweight when diagnosed with stage 2 endometrial cancer. After surgery, it was found that the cancer had spread to one lymph node. Chemotherapy was recommended because she had a very aggressive grade of cancer. She understood that she had to do something about the metabolic syndrome caused by her weight and lack of activity. She managed to adjust her diet and begin to walk for a few minutes a day. Pauline also began a tai chi program, and this made her feel good enough to increase her walking each day. Fortunately, Pauline considered the cancer a wake-up call. She changed her lifestyle completely and is now free of the metabolic syndrome and the visceral fat that had been discovered before her surgery. She has had no further metastasis.

Qigong

Qigong is not so much an exercise as a meditation, but we include it here because it involves motion.

Qigong is from two Chinese words: Qi (pronounced *chi*) means energy and gong (pronounced *kung*) means a skill or a practice. Therefore, qigong means a skill or practice of cultivating energy. There are two categories of qigong—internal and external. The internal kind is like meditation with visualizations that guide energy. The external type includes movement with the meditation.

Qigong is famous in China for curing chronic disease and promoting health and has gained fame recently in the treatment of cancer. A study conducted in China suggests that emitted qi from a master damages tumor cells, inhibits their growth, promotes the regenerative function of the lymph system, and increases antitumorigenic function in rats.

It is believed that regular practice of qigong helps cleanse the body of toxins, restores energy, and reduces stress and anxiety. Numerous studies have reported amazing effects on a variety of illnesses. Similar to meditation and massage, qigong has been shown to reduce blood pressure and pulse rate. While growing in popularity, it remains less studied than acupuncture and massage therapy (see chapter 13).

Two organizations in this country can provide more information about qigong and where you can learn it in your area: The Qigong Institute (www.qigonginstitute.org) and Qigong Association of America (www.qi.org).

CANCER TREATMENT can leave you feeling tired and worn out, but even small steps help you maintain your strength and spirit. Don't begin by aiming for a long walk. This will only discourage you, just as an unrealistic diet will discourage you from losing weight. You will think about walking a mile and decide you cannot do it. Perhaps you can't. Not today, but if you just walk for five or ten minutes, that will be a start. You know the saying about taking just one step. Also, you can do some things while seated or even in bed. You can lift light weights to build some strength in your arms.

Here are some more ideas my patients have suggested for getting exercise:

* While in bed, stretch your arms and legs.
* Put some music on the stereo and dance around the house to slow or fast rhythms, depending on how you feel.
* Plan outings with family or friends that involve physical activity like hiking or swimming.
* Use the fitness center or pool in your neighborhood or at your hotel when traveling.
* On your lunch break, walk around your office building.
* If you have a garden, work in it.

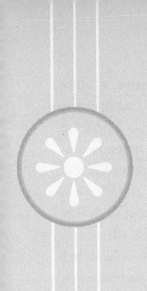

CHAPTER 11

Reducing
the Stress of
Cancer Treatment

IN ADDITION TO THE routine stresses in your life, you now have
the added stress of undergoing cancer treatment. This can affect
you in many ways, depending upon your personality. You may fear
death and become hopeless or helpless. You may fret about losing
your hair or feeling sick. How will cancer treatment affect your job
and your family? If you have a high-stress job, then you may be carrying a heavy burden. This ongoing stress may cause your adrenal
glands to produce excessive cortisol, which in turn boosts your insulin levels. Although most people believe stress impairs their immune system against cancer treatment, the metabolic effect of
stress is far more important.

Stress is not the event or experience but our response to that
event. We all know people who outwardly have little or no stress but
appear on the brink, fearing disaster at every turn. Conversely, some

people seem to experience remarkably traumatic events, whether the loss of a loved one or loss of job or marriage, and maintain the resilience and coping skills to survive. People who experience chronic and unremitting stress often feel they are no longer in control; they don't have the necessary coping mechanisms to adapt and overcome.

Cancer patients bring to their illness the same coping skills that they have used throughout their lives. They may have a large and supportive family and friends to help or they may be isolated and alone, with limited resources to call upon in their time of need. How patients experience their cancer diagnosis may ultimately be as important as the disease itself. A common response to the diagnosis of cancer is to actively fight their disease, mobilizing all their resources in the battle. These patients will seek help from their physicians, exploring both conventional and unconventional treatments in a seemingly relentless fight for survival. Others may placidly accept their diagnosis and let others decide their care. They may seem oblivious to the storm of activity around them, refusing to acknowledge the gravity of their illness. Surprisingly, this "denial" style of coping may be a necessary way of dealing with a dire prognosis. However, when it interferes with early and appropriate medical evaluation or therapy, it can be life threatening.

We all have a degree of control over our lifestyles and there's a lot we can do about relieving chronic stress:

* Seek social support.
* Exercise every day.
* Follow a good diet.
* Choose a form of relaxation, such as meditation, yoga, or prayer, that may generate the "relaxation response" known to dampen down chronic stress.
* Get enough sleep.

Stress can alter your endocrine system by causing abnormal cortisol production and that can prevent medical treatment from working at its best. To get better and stay better you need to get your body and mind in perfect alignment.

There are many ways to lower the stress level, and a variety of these will be suggested in the following chapters with stories of what some of my patients have done. Some reduce stress with massage, while others go out dancing. Some are very good at meditation, guided imagery, and relaxation techniques. Still others gain solace and respite by writing down their thoughts and expressing their emotions in a journal that becomes a growing document reflecting their cancer journey. Most basic to stress reduction must be a personal and individual plan tailored for each person's needs and personality.

There are many programs aimed at helping people reduce stress. For example, some practitioners have patients meditate by striking Tibetan bowls to induce relaxation. Others may provide music or other passive approaches to help patients relax. However, I want my patients to learn how to reduce stress in real life, not just for half an hour of listening to pleasant sounds.

I also help my patients with related health problems such as smoking, weight reduction, and lowering cholesterol as part of the total stress-reduction program. As I have emphasized, many cancer patients remain free of recurrence but are left with the residual effects of their cancer therapy, including increased weight. Coupled with the persistence of fears around their cancer and its recurrence, anxiety and stress remain an issue after treatment is over. As a result, they are also at increased risk of cardiovascular problems and even second cancers. Stress reduction remains an essential part of your well-being well after you have completed cancer treatment.

The Biology of Hope

Integrative practitioners, patients, and the general public pretty much agree that stress has something to do with cancer and its progression. In striking contrast to patients' views, many doctors in the conventional cancer community, while acknowledging the effect of stress on quality of life, dismiss its impact on cancer treatment and its effect on outcomes. Medical research on the role of stress in cancer has been controversial, partly because there has been more focus on the way stress affects the immune system rather than the endocrine system and the metabolic pathways.

It is also understandable that oncologists may not want to generate stress in cancer patients who may be unable to muster the "right attitude." Patients will then likely feel guilty and develop a sense of responsibility for their disease and its outcome. This is dangerous and feeds the sense of helplessness. However, this also reflects a failure by doctors to appreciate the mechanisms through which stress may alter tumor biology. Having cancer is stressful. And that stress has a profound effect on how the body deals with the disease and its treatment.

According to a study reported in *Lancet,* the British medical journal, nonmetastatic breast cancer patients who had a helpless/hopeless or fatalistic mind-set, in contrast to those women with a fighting spirit or who are experiencing denial, had a significantly reduced chance of survival. A high score for depression was also linked to poor outcomes. These effects could not be attributed to other adverse factors such as tumor stage. Sometimes denial and suppression help. In fact, doctors may even provoke hopelessness by crushing a patient's denial. The introduction of psychological therapy can help reduce this hopeless-helpless response.

Avoiding Hopelessness and Helplessness

Many cancer patients feel hopeless and helpless about their disease. They feel hopeless about their chances of survival and helpless to do anything about it. Sometimes these feelings may be unwittingly fostered by the medical community. Many a patient asks the doctor, "What's my prognosis?" When a well-meaning doctor responds by saying, "Forty percent of patients at your stage survive two years," he or she pulls the rug out from under the patient. Or worse, the doctor may say: "Unfortunately, your disease is incurable." While your doctor may often be technically correct, you need to get realistic hope from him or her. Doctors can cure cancer sometimes, improve symptoms and extend life often, and comfort patients always. More important, in the early phases of even advanced cancer, we cannot know how well and for how long a patient's disease can be controlled.

You need to be given realistic hope from your doctor. Here's what that means:

* We can relieve cancer symptoms—always.
* We can extend life—usually.
* We can cure cancer—quite often.

Curing cancer is much more common now, but we need to remember that today's fatal illness is tomorrow's cured disease. We can now keep cancer at bay for longer periods—and this is why we need to feel hope. During that extended period new treatments are being developed. We don't know today what will be available tomorrow.

Hundreds of my patients have proven to me that the "odds" or "percentages" mean nothing when it comes to predicting whether or not one can be cured of cancer. Many of these people have no signs of the advanced cancer they were treated for. Some have a symbiotic relationship with their cancer, keeping it under control with therapy while leading normal lives. One woman who had never smoked had a rare form of cancer in both lungs and was given only months to live. We treated her with Iressa and chemotherapy and she is now moving toward a complete remission. Two years ago, we didn't have that treatment protocol. (Iressa has been replaced by Tarceva, a more effective therapy.)

While most oncologists are increasingly aware of the power of their words, this experience remains all too common. Many of my own patients are with me because they chose to walk rather than remain with a medical practice fostering this sense of hopelessness.

Tom, forty-five, is a graphic artist with metastatic Kaposi's sarcoma to the lung that had developed because he was HIV positive. With another doctor, he had been treated over several months with Adriamycin, a potent form of chemotherapy that left him bald and nauseated much of the time. Despite these side effects, he had only minimal reduction in his tumors and suffered episodes of coughing and breathlessness from the lesions in his lung. A decision was made to withhold further therapy and keep him as comfortable as possible. Tom's disease was hopeless but he was not. He knew he could die but he had the hope to find a physician who would continue trying to cure his disease.

Many people fail to get second opinions, but fortunately Tom wasn't one of them. That's how I met him. One month after this decision, the FDA approved a new class of HIV therapy, protease inhibitors. Rather than start Tom on chemotherapy for the sarcoma, we started him on combination treatment with these new agents to suppress the HIV, and within one month Tom had a 30 percent reduction in his lung tumors. At one year, they had completely resolved and now, four years later, he is active in his work and free of cancer. In contrast to most solid tumors like breast and colon cancer, HIV patients are vulnerable to virally mediated cancers as a result of their immune-deficiency state. By reversing his immune state he was able to unleash his own immune system to reverse the sarcoma and give himself a good future. The immune system in this case is very important.

Mary is another example of hope. At seventy-four she had gastric cancer that caused repeated and sometimes uncontrollable gastrointestinal bleeding. Her doctors recommended that she be placed in hospice care as there were no effective therapies. Fortunately for Mary, her daughter was also a doctor who would not accept this dire prognosis. Mary and her daughter both had hope that Mary would live longer than the few weeks her doctor gave her. Mary had an upper-gastrointestinal endoscope treatment that stopped her bleeding and then underwent several cycles of chemotherapy. Within four weeks she was discharged home, her tumor and liver metastases reduced by 80 percent. With continued chemotherapy and supportive care, including nutrition and selected supplements, Mary had eighteen months of quality life before her disease progressed. In contrast to many patients, neither she nor her physician daughter would accept the dire prognosis that would have afforded her little more than a week or two of survival. While recognizing the ultimate long-term prognosis, she was able to enjoy her family, friends, and many interests, including travel.

As many of my patients have said, "I want to know my doctor *truly believes* that I can do well." Unfortunately, when patients experience this helplessness and hopelessness, the result is an unremitting and excessive stress load with long-term, adverse physiological consequences that may ultimately affect their prognosis.

Insist on Hope from Your Doctors

In dealing with the medical community, insist on hope. Accept nothing less. Unreasonable expectations can lead to inappropriate and often excessive interventions. But an optimistic and hopeful attitude improves the quality of life and blunts the adverse emotional impact of treatment side effects. I have many patients with metastatic cancer whose outcomes have far exceeded expectations of their first treating physicians. In some cases they have left treatment because they felt their doctors did not believe they could do well. Even when patients have progressed and eventually succumbed, despite our best and continued efforts to support them emotionally, no family member has ever said, "I'm sorry you gave her hope."

Realistic hopefulness is one of our most powerful allies and effective stress busters, particularly when supported by your own doctor. In an early study of integrative cancer treatments from England in the 1980s, patients were very satisfied with the use of complementary therapies along with conventional care. They understood that there may be little effect on tumor progression and outcome but the hope it provided them was of great value. Study after study indicates that, for most patients, it is the doctor's words, not those of other health-care providers assisting them, that carry the most emotional weight. As I have frequently told our medical residents in training, the words of the physician are more powerful than the scalpel of the surgeon.

Jeanette has breast cancer and was told by her physician that she had a 45 percent chance of cure. By doing this, the doctor crushed her hope for the future. With the encouragement of her family and friends, she wisely came for a second opinion and is doing just fine with treatment and support. Because of the rapidly changing nature of adjuvant breast cancer therapy, I was able to provide her with realistic hope for a healthy future. She had a large tumor that had spread beyond the breast to two lymph nodes under her arm. Because she is several years past menopause, I suggested an aggressive dose-dense regimen with three chemotherapy drugs: Adriamycin, Cytoxan, and Taxol, to be followed by radiation. When she completed chemotherapy and radiation, she began hormonal therapy with an aromatase inhibitor that blocks estrogen production within the fatty tissue. We have no long-term proof yet that these agents will prevent recurrence of her cancer. But twenty years ago we had no long-term proof about tamoxifen either. Today, we know that it prevents recurrence of breast cancer. With constant additions to our conventional medicine cabinet, we can continue to reduce risk of cancer recurrence and death.

Advocate for Better Care

One of my patients is a great example of how having hope for yourself and advocating for better care for others can help the patient, too. Mark not only didn't lose hope for himself, but helped others gain the same feeling.

Mark was only moderately overweight, but his excess weight was a spare tire around his middle. His waist size had ballooned to forty-two from thirty-six inches over the last ten years. At sixty-eight, he had been in a stressful executive job, had recently developed high blood pressure, and now had a newly diagnosed pancreatic cancer. His cancer had spread to the liver, so we could not cure it with surgical removal of the pancreas. In addition to his routine staging and pretreatment testing, he was evaluated for evidence of insulin resistance. Blood tests revealed high fasting levels of insulin and C-peptide (a measure of ongoing insulin secretion by the pancreas), high circulating triglycerides, and a low percentage of the good cholesterol (HDL, or high-density lipoproteins) in his blood.

He began a conventional chemotherapy regimen with gemcitabine for his pancreatic cancer and a program of nutrition and selected supplements for weight reduction. He also began to change his lifestyle to reduce stress with daily meditation and a moderate exercise program.

Mark's greatest source of solace and support came from his own efforts to start an informal program to assist other cancer patients. He became a vigorous advocate of active patient involvement in their own care, encouraging them to follow his path of diet and exercise. He was a crucial example of hope and connectedness that patients long for. After months of treatment, his pancreatic cancer had shrunk to 20 percent of its original size and the liver metastases had disappeared.

Mark had been off chemotherapy and feeling good for six months when his tumor showed evidence of regrowth. He simultaneously had signs of a rising insulin level. After restarting chemotherapy and redoubling efforts at reducing insulin resistance, he has had a dramatic shrinkage in both his pancreatic tumor and the metastatic liver lesions. He continues to be well and free of cancer symptoms nearly three years after his original diagnosis.

While chemotherapy has been absolutely necessary in Mark's case, by reducing his insulin-resistant state through diet and exercise, we believe his treatment has been more effective. He also made important changes that helped limit his stressful lifestyle. While cognizant of the serious implications of his cancer, his hopeful outlook has helped him through the rigors of chemotherapy and provided an example of what is possible for his fellow patients.

Cancer Is Not a Hopeless Disease

These cases illustrate the difficulty of giving a prognosis today for tomorrow it may quickly change. Hope is not misleading. It is essential.

Hope is necessary to successful treatment of cancer. If you lose hope, the risk increases for stress-related changes that impact the outcome of treatment. There's a true biological basis to hope. When we take away hope, it essentially begins the dying process. If patients are strong and unusual, they will rebel and quickly seek other doctors or treatment. They choose to walk rather than remain with doctors who foster such hopelessness.

Dr. D. S. Sobel, from the regional health education department of Kaiser Permanente Medical Program in California, said this: "Thoughts, feelings, and moods may have significant effects on the onset, course, and outcome of many diseases. By helping patients manage not just their disease but also common underlying needs for psychological support, coping skills, and sense of control, health outcomes can be significantly improved in a cost-effective manner."

Cancer is not a hopeless disease. There are more than ten million survivors in this country to prove that.

Building a Social Support Network

A support network is essential. One of the most important ways to reduce stress is to maximize your social connections.

A study from Yale University followed African-American and white women with newly diagnosed breast cancer for ten years. The psychological factor most predictive of survival was the presence of "perceived social support." The women were asked whether they could talk about cancer freely with friends and relatives. Those who could not had a shorter survival.

In a similar study from the California Department of Health Services, women with the lowest number of reported close friends and relatives had the highest breast cancer death rates. Women in Australia with newly diagnosed breast cancer who had severe and multiple stressors had poor outcomes. However, when they had two or more active caregivers, this stress effect disappeared.

Strong emotional support from friends or family is a powerful stress-buster for cancer patients. Asking your friends and family to pitch in and go for a walk with you or relieve you of some stressful chores also helps them. People who volunteer show fewer symptoms of stress, as helping others gives a sense of purpose.

Our own chemotherapy treatment room is a hubbub of activity. Patients are encouraged to come with one or more friends or relatives. Despite often prolonged chemotherapy treatments that may last up to eight hours, there is a constant hum of conversation and laughter. One of our "elder statesman" patients frequently regales the crew with jokes and gags. There is an abundance of home-cooked foods, sometimes goodies to reward patients at the end of a long day. None of the chairs are segregated in separate, isolating cubicles and patients have expressed their desire to keep it this way, though all are offered the option of being treated privately, in a separate room with a comfortable chair and relaxing, tranquil view.

I can feel it the minute I walk into my office. I feel the warmth and caring and most surprisingly, the laughter coming from my patients undergoing chemotherapy. I am administering the treatment in a group setting while patients are talking to one another, having, in effect, established their own support group.

This group setting, with its own spontaneous and ever-changing support-group atmosphere, is called healing and nurturing by many of the patients and reflects their need to connect. While aspects of illness are frequently discussed, the conversation almost always returns to nonmedical talk. One patient was overheard saying, "I look forward to my chemo day every week."

Cancer Support Groups

Support groups, though not necessarily for everyone, play a major role in complementary cancer therapy. The classic 1989 Stanford University study by David Spiegel, using group psychotherapy in eighty-six women with metastatic breast cancer, unexpectedly demonstrated a marked improvement in survival. While a recent multi-center trial modeled after the original failed to show the same survival effect, support groups clearly benefited mood and quality of life in participants. In this newer study, it may have been impossible to provide an adequate "control" group because family and community support have become commonplace in the years since the original study.

One of the most important developments in cancer care over the last twenty years has been the growing network of cancer support groups. Virtually every community and academic cancer center provides support groups, where you can find invaluable sources of information about cancer treatments, effective options for dealing with treatment side effects, and, most important, a network for cancer patients to share experiences and connect in a safe setting.

For some cancer patients, this is the only social connection. They would otherwise be alone and isolated. A newer phenomenon is the Internet support group that allows homebound patients to connect to others. Many of these support groups devote time to psychological interventions aimed at ameliorating the stress of cancer.

Be sure to ask your doctors, nurses, anyone involved in your care about support groups. There are also sources listed on the Internet. Check the American Cancer Society and specific cancer groups such as the Breast Cancer Alliance.

Stress-Reduction Program for Caregivers

Family caregivers provide the bulk of care to cancer patients and suffer significant adverse health impacts, both emotionally and physically. In my practice, we have a program that gives the families of our patients information and lifestyle coping skills to maximize their health and reduce any health impact of the caregiver's stress while optimizing their real and perceived efficiency.

This is multidisciplinary but based on a mind-body skills program. It includes meditation, stress-management techniques with informational materials, as well as massage and other relaxation techniques. Sleep deprivation and its consequences—much like the stress of caring for cancer patients themselves—increase caregivers' risk for a variety of chronic illnesses, as well as a significant social and job disruption with resulting financial hardship. Because cancer is a disease involving not just an individual but involving their entire extended family, stress reduction is a family issue. The effective caregiver must also be cared for.

One woman came from another part of the country to care for her sister in a New York hospital during her cancer treatment. She spent all day or all night in the hospital, alternating with her sister's husband, so that one of them was always at her bedside. Sometimes the sister stayed around the clock for two or three days. One day she fainted and had to be admitted to the hospital herself. She had lupus as well as a thyroid condition. And while these conditions had been under control for years, the stress caught up with her. The ill woman's husband also ended up in the hospital because his blood pressure had skyrocketed, so his normal medications were not working. These two are examples of what happens when you don't deal with the stress of caregiving for a seriously ill cancer patient. Had they made sure to eat well, exercise every day, and practice some stress-relieving techniques, they might have been able to avoid their own illnesses.

There are many family caregiver organizations that have programs and other resources. You can contact the National Cancer Institute and the American Cancer Society to find such programs in your area, but here are some of them:

* Family Caregiver Alliance (www.caregiver.org)
* National Alliance for Caregiving (www.caregiving.org)
* National Family Caregivers Association (www.thefamilycaregiver.org)
* Well Spouse Foundation (www.wellspouse.org)

Having cancer is stressful. Even the strongest, most optimistic person needs to acknowledge this. If you consider the treatment of the stress as a necessary part of your overall cancer therapy, then you will not only feel better, your cancer treatment will be more effective. Avail yourself of all the tools you can to achieve this goal.

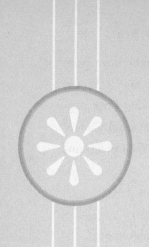

Using the Power
of Your Mind
to Ease the Stress
of Cancer Treatment

WHILE YOU ARE BEING treated for cancer your body is being attacked by drugs, radiation, or surgery. During the months of therapy while your body is under siege, you need to use the power of your mind to help your body deal with this stress. There are ways to do this with guided imagery, progressive muscle relaxation, meditation, and hypnosis. There are ways to get your body ready for surgery so that you will recover more quickly. Remember what we said earlier: in order to heal, you need your body and mind in perfect alignment.

These mind-body techniques have many benefits:

* Decreased levels of stress
* Increased immune functioning
* Decreased pain
* Faster recovery from procedures

✳ Fewer side effects from chemotherapy

✳ Less anticipatory nausea and vomiting before chemotherapy

✳ Decreased anxiety

✳ Improved mood and less suppression of emotions

Relaxation also helps you gain perspective on every aspect of your life, and to feel less overwhelmed by the cancer and treatment. If you can relax during a difficult time, it is, by definition, no longer such a powerful stressor to you. My goal is to provide techniques based on my patients' own interest and affinity to help them cope with conventional treatment as well as improving recovery after completing treatment. The additional benefit of normalizing cortisol rhythms, and, with that, limiting excessive insulin and other metabolic mediators of cancer growth, may limit cancer recurrence and tumor growth.

The More You Know, the Better You Can Cope

The first step in coping with your condition healthily is to determine exactly where you stand with your cancer and its treatment. If you are plagued by doubts, you will not be able to relax enough to get rid of the stress. There is a program called The Facts and Coping developed by Georgetown University Center for Mind-Body Medicine. This simply means that the more you know, the better you can cope. This is true of any situation, but especially of cancer. In my practice, we describe the nature of the particular cancer a person has and how it works in their body. Patients who are educated in this way are better able to come to grips with the disease. It helps get rid of myths and hearsay that may be adding to their anxiety level. Once they can put their disease in its proper perspective, understand how aggressive—or not—their cancer is, and how it will affect their body and their lifestyle, they can make plans for the best ways to adapt and work toward getting better.

Melanie was diagnosed with breast cancer shortly after the birth of her second child. At forty she was a stay-at-home mom. Despite having a small cancer and no lymph-node involvement, we believed she needed chemotherapy after surgery because breast cancer in young women tends to be aggressive. At our first meeting, Melanie expressed extreme fear and anxiety over her future. She had a very supportive husband and family but remained preoccupied with a fear of dying. She was unable to sleep and prior to her first chemotherapy session she was nauseated.

Carefully exploring her fears, we found that a childhood friend's mother had died of breast cancer when Melanie and her friend were ten years old. Being a young mother heightened her sense of vulnerability and that of her family. She was reluctant to share this even with her husband, partly from fear of her own prognosis. With the help of a social worker trained in cancer support and a stress-reduction specialist, we were able to address Melanie's fears and support her through chemotherapy. Left unaddressed, the toll on her emotionally and physically was unpredictable.

Learn all you can about your cancer and its treatment. Talk with your doctor and ask questions until you feel confident. There is a great deal of health information available today through books like this one and through the Internet. Make sure you contact reputable online sources, however, such as the National Cancer Institute.

Relaxing Your Breathing

Breathing deeply and slowly maximizes the flow of oxygen into the blood, which promotes a sense of relaxation. Try this: inhale fully, paying attention to your stomach's rise and fall. To shift from chest breathing to abdominal breathing, make one or two full exhalations to push out air from the bottom of the lungs, which allows for an abdominal breath on the next slow inhalation.

Progressive Muscle Relaxation

Progressive muscle relaxation means focusing on sequential muscle groups, relaxing the tension as you move from one area to another. If you begin with your feet, you think about your toes, focus on relaxing those muscles, work up toward your ankle, your calf, knee, and so on until you reach your head. Or, you can start with your head and work down.

Finding a Quiet Place

Your environment plays a big role in helping you relax. For example, it would be difficult to relax completely in a noisy busy office or a part of your home that is constantly filled with other people. You need a quiet place without interruption where you feel safe. Perhaps there's a room in your home conducive to relaxation. Pastels can have a calming effect, and some interior decorators claim that greens and blues promote relaxation. Or with guided imagery (see below), you can imagine that place. Think of the calming effect of staring into the blue ocean or looking at an endless field of green. If you have access to that field or ocean, by all means go there!

Guided Imagery

Guided imagery is the use of mental images to help you influence how your body feels. That is, training your imagination to bring you to a less stressful place. Not everybody is visually oriented to the same degree. Artists, for example, clearly see images in their minds. They can see the landscape or people or picture an entire action movie. In fact, the mental imagery can be so real that they can be confused about whether or not they actually experienced the scene. Other people may need some help in developing this ability. Think of this as making movies in your mind.

Your thoughts and the images that flow from your imagination influence your emotions and spirit as well as your body. Your brain doesn't always know if you are actually experiencing what you are thinking about. Just think of all the multitasking we do these days. People seem able to operate a computer, talk on the phone, and make a grocery list all at once. We are all capable of worrying over something and thinking the worst. For instance, a person who is afraid to fly will always picture the plane crashing. But if the desire to get to Paris, say, is stronger, that person can learn to change the pictures. By picturing herself happily touring the Eiffel Tower, the picture (and fear) of the plane crashing will diminish.

It's the same with cancer treatment. Picture yourself feeling relaxed and your body responding to treatment. You can learn to use this kind of power to produce calming and healing responses in your body. Rather than random thinking about your cancer treatment and your stress and fears, guided imagery can help you channel your imagination into a constructive part of your therapy. Think of it as controlled daydreaming.

You can learn these techniques by using them daily or at least three times a week. Guided imagery can be used to reduce anxiety, decrease muscle tension and pain, ease sleep problems, speed healing and recovery from surgery, and last but not least, give you a sense of mastery and control.

The psychological benefits of guided imagery have been documented in many studies. Common guided-imagery techniques use positive mental images such as immune cells attacking the cancer.

If you remember pop culture of the 1980s, you can picture the video Pac-Man gobbling up cancer cells.

Some of these approaches use a process well known to psychologists as restructuring. You learn to replace an anticipated, unpleasant symptom or emotion with an image of the opposite effect. Let's say you fear getting so sick from chemotherapy that just thinking about that could make you feel nauseated. So try to replace that fearful image with one of breathing deeply in a safe place until the nausea passes. This may not sound easy, but with practice it can be done by anyone, and it works.

You will be encouraged to create your own image, such as feeling comfortable, relaxed, and pain free in a remembered safe place when undergoing a traumatic or painful medical procedure in the hospital. Similarly, by evoking memories of pleasant sensations, you can reduce anticipatory nausea before you begin chemotherapy.

Special-place imagery reduces stress and anxiety, increases relaxation, and strengthens your capacity to draw on your own emotional resources. This technique provides a foundation for other imagery exercises. It can also provoke strong emotional memories.

In my practice we work with the guided-imagery program designed by the Georgetown University Center for Mind and Body Medicine. Here's how it works:

Sit back and relax. Loosen any clothing that feels tight. Remove your glasses if you wish and see that your arms and legs are in a position that feels right for you. Once you are comfortable, slowly and gently close your eyes. Allow your attention to move to your breathing. Let it become even and comfortable. Breathing is one of the most powerful conscious influences you have on your nervous system.

Now see yourself in a very special place. It could be a real place, someplace you've been, perhaps a beautiful spot in nature, a beach or garden, or a comforting place in your own home. You can also visit an imaginary place, indoors or outdoors, perhaps something from a story or movie. If more than one place comes to mind, try to stay with just one.

All that matters is that it is a place where you feel perfectly safe and comfortable. Appreciate this scene with all of your senses. Hear the sounds, smell the aromas, feel the air as it caresses your skin. Try to experience the ground securely under you. Touch and feel the whole environment. Begin to notice things. What are you wearing? What is on your feet? What time of year and day is it? How old are you? Are you alone or with other people? Is it warm or cold? As you experience this environment, think about what else would make this place safe for you. Maybe you need to add or remove something. Notice how your body feels. Enjoy this feeling of safety in your special place. Once you are ready, you can visit this place whenever you want. When you are ready, let your breathing deepen. Gradually feel your body against the chair again. Bring yourself back slowly. Notice how good you feel.

Guided imagery played an important role for Bill, fifty-six, who was referred to me with progressive high-grade prostate cancer. The cancer was confined to the prostate, and he had been stable until six months before he came to see me when his PSA went to 60 and the bone scan showed signs of cancer invasion. However, the CT showed no other organ involvement. During this time he had gained fifteen pounds and was thirty pounds over his weight from fifteen years ago. His triglycerides, blood, and C-peptides were high. Bill ate poorly and did little exercise, so we planned an aggressive lifestyle change including a low-calorie diet, vigorous aerobic exercise, weight training, and a stress-reduction program with meditation and guided imagery. Bill agreed to hormone therapy with Zoladex, and a bisphosphonate called Zometa (zoledronic acid) to reduce his bone metastasis. Now, three months into treatment, his weight is down ten pounds and his PSA is normalizing and only slightly elevated. This shows the importance of an integrative approach in maximizing cancer treatment.

There are many places to find information about guided imagery and get tapes, DVDs, and books to help you learn:

* Georgetown University Center for Mind and Body Medicine: www.cmbm.org
* The Academy for Guided Imagery at www.academyfor guidedimagery.com
* InnerVision Studio, Inc. at www.innervisionstudioinc.com
* CancerImagery.com at www.cancerimagery.com

Reducing the Stress of Surgery

Fear is the feeling most commonly reported by people about to undergo surgery. They fear the unknown, fear a change in body image, fear death, disability, pain, or poor prognosis, as well as fear powerlessness. Such stress can undermine your body at a time when you need it to help heal you.

Doctors prepare you for the mechanical aspects of surgery, explaining what will happen to your body. They may not realize how frightening that can sound, so you need to know how to put your mind and body in the proper state for best results.

You can do this using a program by Peggy Huddleston called Prepare for Surgery, Heal Faster (www.healfaster.com). It includes a brief but comprehensive stress reduction program to reduce your anxiety before surgery and the pain after surgery, as well as hasten recovery.

Huddleston's five steps, briefly:

1. Relax to feel peaceful.
2. Visualize your healing.
3. Organize a support group.

4.   Use healing statements.
5.   Meet your anesthesiologist.

This program has been shown to reduce postoperative pain and shorten the recovery time. It is particularly beneficial for patients who have never undergone surgery or have superimposed stress and anxiety from a cancer diagnosis and are having a definitive cancer operation. It helps calm the jitters. Feeling peaceful strengthens your immune system and creates the complex biochemistry that enhances healing.

A one-and-a-half to two-hour session, either individually or with a group, is based on guided imagery and cognitive restructuring techniques. You talk about your fears and reframe those fears into healing and comforting images. You can record these thoughts on tape and listen to them before surgery and while you recover.

There are commercially prepared tapes with healing statements for those who feel shy about making their own. You can get these tapes from www.healfaster.com. This is followed by a meeting with the anesthesiologists just before and right after surgery. The anesthesiologist is asked to repeat the healing statements as you are being initially sedated for surgery. This reinforces the effect. While some are skeptical, anesthesiologists understand the anxiety surrounding any surgical procedure and usually welcome the chance to help reduce a patient's anxiety and the need for postoperative pain medication. You recover quicker, too. By visualizing your recovery, you turn worries into healing imagery. You learn how to surround yourself in love of family and friends to calm yourself before surgery.

In a study of chemotherapy-specific guided-imagery audiotape, those using the tape had a more positive experience with their chemotherapy. A study from Hadassah University Hospital in Israel compared patients with localized cancer using progressive muscle relaxation and guided imagery with a control group that did not.

Those using the tape had less overall psychological distress. (The study also suggested that the benefits would have been greater if it had excluded those patients who already had a low level of distress.)

I recommend using a relaxation tape every day for two weeks before surgery. The tapes are often used on the way to the operating room to reduce the anticipatory fear. Many have also found this valuable after surgery to reduce pain and speed recovery. This is an effective stress-reducing technique in preparation for chemotherapy to reduce the anticipatory nausea.

Paul, a retired lawyer, was diagnosed with lung cancer after a persistent respiratory infection failed to resolve with antibiotics. Tests revealed a large mass in his right lung, but the cancer had not spread outside of the lung. In anticipation of removal of his lung, Paul participated in the pre-op relaxation program in our office. He went to surgery using the tape with help from the anesthesiologist. Despite this extensive operation, and to the surprise of the surgical nursing staff, Paul was breathing on his own within twenty-four hours, out of bed and walking the hallway by his third day, and was discharged one day later. Another patient, operated on the same day with a less extensive operation but without the pre-op preparation, remained in the hospital three days longer than Paul. Paul attributed his remarkable recovery to the sense of peace and relaxation he gained from continuing to listen to his pre-op relaxation tape during his recovery. When he started on post-op chemotherapy, he again used his tape to prepare himself for the anticipated side effects.

Using healing statements, words that are spoken during surgery, can reduce the use of pain medication by up to 50 percent.

Meditation

The power of the mind to influence bodily function has long been of interest to scientists, reflecting the growing recognition of connections between the nervous, immune, and endocrine systems. Scientific research in the United States has focused on the short-term effects of meditation, finding that it reduces markers of stress like heart rate and perspiration. Among the first to study the physiological effects of Zen meditation, Dr. Herbert Benson of the Harvard Center for Mind-Body Medicine has documented the relaxation response, a deep autonomic response to meditation, in his book *The Relaxation Response*. He has demonstrated many clinical settings where meditation may have benefits, including pain control, hypertension, infertility, reduced anxiety, and reduced nausea from chemotherapy.

Jon Kabat-Zinn has pioneered meditation in the medical setting, too, with his Mindfulness Based Stress Reduction program (MBSR). Since founding the stress-reduction clinic at the University of Massachusetts Medical School in 1979, Kabat-Zinn and colleagues have treated patients and taught health professionals the techniques of mindfulness meditation. There are some intriguing studies showing that cancer patients who practiced meditation had significantly better emotional outlooks than a control group.

Once the exclusive province of Eastern religious traditions, meditation is now valued for relaxation and stress reduction by people around the world. Many medically based meditation programs have been studied in the setting of chronic illness.

Buddhist meditation emphasizes enduring changes in mental activity, not just short-term results. Some studies suggest that many meditation techniques may have not only emotional effects but also distinct physiological effects. That is, the power of meditation might be harnessed in a way that not only reduces stress and defuses negative emotion, but improves immune function, reduces blood pressure, and affects numerous other systems in a beneficial way.

Using Kabat-Zinn's MBSR program, researchers at the Alberta Cancer Board have evaluated its benefits in patients with breast and prostate cancer. People enrolled in the program reduced stress and improved the quality of life.

That meditation has any effect on tumor progression remains unproven. However, a small study of men with a rising PSA after prostate surgery (a harbinger of cancer recurrence) on a low-fat, high-fiber diet was combined with such a meditation program for four months. Most of the men showed a decrease in the rate of rise of the PSA and several had a decline in number. It took PSA levels nearly eighteen months rather than the usual six and a half months to double after surgery.

Studies at the University of California at San Diego and the University of Massachusetts looked at men combining mindfulness stress reduction with a low-fat, high-fiber plant diet and the effect on PSA levels after surgery. The men who meditated and followed their diet showed a decline in rate of rise of PSA. Thus, the rate of recurrence is slowed.

Many meditation practices are available, the simplest being to focus on your breathing, allowing your random thoughts to relax control over your conscious state. One of the most effective and practical meditation practices is a form of walking meditation known as BreathWalk (see chapter 10). This technique combines the conscious focus on the specific pattern or breathing synchronized with our walking steps. By learning first how to breathe in a healthy pattern and then combining it with walking rhythm, we develop a valuable way to generate relaxation response while simultaneously getting exercise. It is particularly beneficial when practiced with a group of friends or fellow patients. Documented benefits have included improved mood and sense of well-being, increased energy level, and a sense of connectedness.

For more information, look for *The Relaxation Response* by Dr. Herbert Benson and Jon Kabat-Zinn's *Full Catastrophe Living: Using the Wisdom of Your Mind to Face Stress, Pain, and Illness.*

Other resources providing how-to information and other links on meditation are:

www.Wildmind.org

www.ananda.org

www.buddhamind.info

Individual Hypnosis

Hypnosis is a very valuable and common tool used by medical professionals in one-on-one situations. It works for smoking cessation and many stress-related behaviors. It can often be used with guided imagery.

Beginning hypnosis before chemotherapy is a way to help patients who have an anticipatory anxiety about feeling sick after treatment. One woman developed nausea in the treatment room before she got chemotherapy. It was a conditioned reflex before her first injection. She got so sick that we had to get psychological help for her. The hypnosis worked for her—after a few sessions, she was able to get on with her chemotherapy treatment. The nausea she had so feared never occurred.

WHEN THE mind and body are in harmony, treatment is more effective. Continuing these techniques after the end of treatment will help you keep your life and health in harmony every day for the rest of your life.

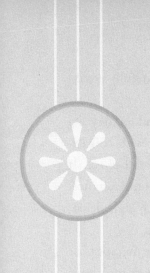

CHAPTER 13

Massage Therapy and Other Bodywork

HUMAN TOUCH IS ESSENTIAL to our long-term well-being. We've long known that massage helps premature babies survive. At the Touch Research Institute at the University of Miami School of Medicine, the medical benefits of massage were documented in many situations, including cancer.

Some oncology hospital units, including my own, have a licensed medical massage therapist on staff. Our pilot study showed a significant reduction in anxiety and a mild reduction in pain in cancer patients receiving massage. One of our first patients was a sixty-four-year-old woman with breast cancer that spread to her bones. When she came to the hospital, she had not slept for two weeks because of bone pain. That evening she was given a gentle one-hour massage with cautions because of her bone metastasis.

She had a sound and restful sleep that night and gratefully attributed it to the relaxation she felt after the massage.

Licensed massage therapists help relieve stress and anxiety before and after a patient's chemotherapy. In concert with conventional medical treatment, this can enhance the overall effect. It helps reduce stress in those with stress-related insulin resistance. And manual lymphatic massage helps patients with lymphedema, swelling caused by blockage in lymphatic circulation.

In some studies, massage either by trained massage therapists or nurses trained in massage techniques may help in short-term pain relief. This may partly reflect an improvement in anxiety and a consequent rise in pain thresholds.

Massage can improve the function of the immune, endocrine, and nervous systems. It also lowers blood pressure, pulse, and respiratory rate, all reflections of the relaxation response. Virtually all studies indicate an improvement in the sense of well-being and quality of life for most patients.

In my practice we also offer massage for the family caregivers of our cancer patients, who experience the enormous stress of caring for loved ones with chronic illness. The medical as well as psychological benefits are not without substance, given the increase in illness risk in this group, which faces difficulty and frustration and sometimes hopelessness.

Chinese Massage

Chinese massage is effective for a range of health problems and it is widely practiced and taught in hospitals and medical schools. It is an essential part of primary health care in China and many other countries. Chinese massage encompasses five related and overlapping techniques including: press and rub; push and grasp; and point press. Like acupuncture, it focuses on a system of pathways that transport energy through the body. In traditional Chinese medicine, pain is viewed as simply a lack of free flow of qi (the body's energy; also spelled chi) and blood and this is why Chinese massage is such a powerful treatment for pain. It uses a system of gentle and soft yet deep and penetrating techniques. Strokes are applied with rhythm and persistence. It is almost always given through the clothing on a couch or a stool. However, it can be done directly on the skin.

Reflexology

The ancient art of reflexology was first practiced by the early Indian, Chinese, and Egyptian peoples. It involves the use of hands to apply gentle pressure to the feet. Trained hands can detect tiny deposits and imbalances in the feet and by working on these points the reflexologist can release blockages and restore the free flow of energy to the whole body. Tension is eased, circulation is improved. This encourages the body to heal itself at its own pace. A session might take an hour or just five or ten minutes. Increasingly, reflexology is being used in hospitals to treat cancer patients.

* Ongoing studies at the University of Liverpool in England revealed that reflexology improved the quality of life.

* In Australia, the introduction of a simple and safe foot massage by nurses in hospitalized cancer patients, for five minutes per foot, significantly reduced nausea and pain and produced a relaxed state. A similar program for breast and lung cancer patients decreased anxiety and reduced pain in a third of patients.

* In the United States, researchers at the School of Nursing, East Carolina University, in North Carolina, found that foot reflexology alleviated anxiety and pain for twenty-three patients with breast and lung cancer.

＊ Many other studies around the world have found that the practice not only eases anxiety and pain, but halves some treatment side effects, such as nausea.

Reflexology is one of many integrative-care practices now used at cancer centers. *The American Cancer Society Journal* in 1998 found that one third of cancer patients used reflexology. The American College of Physicians and American Society of Internal Medicine Web page currently advocates the learning and use of reflexology in a home-care guide for advanced cancer.

Acupuncture and Acupressure

These similar techniques help reduce nausea from chemotherapy, reduce stress and pain, and also help patients quit smoking. (We have ongoing studies on chemotherapy and cancer-related fatigue in progress and available to our patients.)

Acupuncture is an ancient Chinese therapeutic process in which specific points of the body are stimulated with needles to foster healing or pain relief. The theory is that the body's energy—qi, or chi—is carried along pathways called meridians. When you are ill, the flow of chi in the twelve primary meridians is out of synch. By stimulating specific points along the meridians, the flow can be corrected to optimize health or block pain. Western researchers theorize that in cases where acupuncture eases pain, it does so by stimulating the central nervous system to release chemicals (endorphins) that lessen the *perception* of pain. (Acupressure uses pressure rather than needles on the same meridians.)

Thin needles are used at the 360 specific points along the meridians. As few as five, or as many as fifteen, sterile needles are inserted from a mere fraction of an inch to four inches deep. As the needles are inserted, you may feel a light needle prick to tingling, warmth, or pinching. The needles are left in place from five to sixty minutes (twenty minutes is about the average). A course of ten treatments is usually needed to obtain maximum benefit. Follow-up treatments, usually every few months, are advised to maintain normal energy balance. Some therapists may use heat, pressure, friction, suction, or electrical current—in addition to needles or in place of them.

However it works, acupuncture has a role in managing short-term acute pain. While it seems to have some benefit for the treatment of certain chronic pain, there is no evidence yet that it is effective for long-term pain. Theoretically, acupuncture could relieve significant pain of various origins for at least a short time, just as it has been used to control pain during surgery in China.

The National Institutes of Health reviewed data on acupuncture and confirmed the benefit in various settings, including pain and chemotherapy-related nausea. Nausea was either reduced or prevented in 97 percent of patients with no side effects from the acupuncture.

While control of nausea and pain in cancer patients has been well documented, acupuncture may have other benefits as well. Studies show a dramatic improvement in the debilitating side effect from radiation for head and neck cancer, called xerostomia. This is a profound decrease in saliva production accompanied by dry mouth, oral discomfort, and impaired swallowing. Acupuncture improves salivary flow significantly and reduces symptoms. A limited number of trials suggest that hot flashes from breast cancer hormone treatments and prostate cancer hormonal ablation may be reduced with acupuncture treatment, but more research is needed.

Acupuncture is something to consider if medications cannot be used to combat the toxic side effects of chemotherapy. However, it is a passive, time-consuming procedure that is not yet universally covered by medical insurance.

Acupuncture has a good safety record when it's done by a licensed practitioner using universal precautions. However, there are possible complications, such as infections (AIDS or hepatitis), if sterile needles are not used. Theoretically, organs may be punctured and local bleeding may occur, causing a large bruise, especially for patients on blood thinners such as aspirin or other nonsteroidal anti-inflammatory drugs (NSAIDs), or worse, Coumadin.

Acupuncture was crucial to the survival of Henry, fifty-five, a bartender. Although he doesn't drink excessively, he did smoke two packs of cigarettes a day. Even when the no-smoking laws arrived in most bars in New York City, Henry managed to smoke on his breaks and then smoked even more when outside of his work environment. He was not overweight, but had a sizeable pot belly. He also suffered from what he thought was indigestion and was constantly popping Tums and other antacids. To top it all off, Henry did no exercise except for walking back and forth behind the bar, which actually caused him quite a bit of stress because he was standing all the time but unable to stretch his muscles. When his so-called indigestion got so bad he began to have excruciating pain, he went to the doctor. He was diagnosed with esophageal cancer and went into surgery. Fortunately, his cancer had not spread and surgery was curative. However, he had also been diagnosed with the metabolic syndrome and was in a prediabetic state. Dietary changes, exercise, and smoking cessation were highly recommended.

Acupuncture helped him stop smoking, and he joined a group therapy class to learn how to reduce stress. He now goes to a gym before he goes to work, eats nutritious regular meals—no more high-calorie bar food—and feels better than he has in years. Without that dangerous fat around his middle, his tests reveal that the metabolic syndrome is no longer a risk for Henry.

Many of our patients have noted a significant improvement in energy and sense of well-being and continue their acupuncture treatment well beyond their cancer treatments.

Do-It-Yourself Acupressure

Acupressure involves the same specific meridian points on the body, but rather than using needles to stimulate them, practitioners use their hands. They apply pressure with fingers, knuckles, and the palms of their hands. It probably evolved out of the natural human instinct to hold or rub a part of the body that hurts. Acupressure actually predates acupuncture by more than two thousand years. While the Chinese typically use acupressure as a first-aid treatment on themselves and family members, in America it is used primarily to relieve pain and reduce stress. A trained therapist can teach you the techniques, but you can learn to perform acupressure on your own body.

You can focus continuously on one particular pain meridian. This is something like the patient-controlled analgesia used in hospital settings, where the patient pushes a button to get more pain medication when needed.

To reduce the nausea caused by cancer treatment, you can apply an elasticized wrist band over the acupressure site—the P6 meridian on the wrist. This site controls nausea and should be pressed every two hours. The antinausea effect could be prolonged for up to twenty-four hours. Visit an acupressure therapist to learn how to do this before you try. Some other cautions about do-it-yourself acupressure include:

* Never press on an open wound or any area that is swollen or inflamed.
* Don't press on the area over a tumor.
* Don't press on the area directly over lymph nodes.

Reiki

Reiki is a holistic healing art that originated in ancient Tibet. It's a hands-on technique that gently helps restore balance to the body, mind, and spirit. The word Reiki means universal life energy (rei) brought through personal energy (ki). Reiki is used to promote relaxation, reduce stress, and accelerate the body's natural ability to heal from physical ailments.

A Reiki session usually lasts twenty minutes as the practitioner directs healing energy to the recipient's body. It is a collaborative exchange. The practitioner provides a channel for the flow of energy, which will be used by the recipient in their healing process. Therefore, the recipient's willingness and open attitude during treatment influences the amount of Reiki energy received, and progress is made.

Jason had metastatic colon cancer and was debilitated by severe peripheral neuropathy (nerve pain) because he was also diabetic. Despite improved glucose control with diet and activity treatment for his pain, he had limited ability to exercise because of his constant discomfort. We started him on Reiki treatments several days a week and within one month Jason felt well enough to restart his exercise program. When he missed his Reiki treatment, however, his symptoms returned. We still don't understand the mechanism of action. It could be a powerful placebo effect from the relationship with the practitioner. There are no adverse effects and Reiki can enhance symptom control. It cannot—as is true of all complementary treatments—serve as an alternative to effective conventional medical care.

THESE PHYSICAL techniques for easing stress and helping reduce pain could be categorized as "hands-on medicine."

Whichever one, or even more than one of these techniques, works best for you, try to make it part of your overall cancer therapy. If therapists are not available at your cancer treatment center, ask your doctor and other health-care practitioners for recommendations.

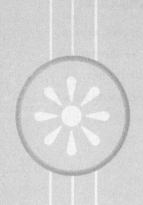

CHAPTER 14

How to Sleep
with Cancer

IT IS IMPOSSIBLE to get a good night's sleep in a hospital. Doctors make their rounds and wake up people at 5 or 6 A.M., disrupting their sleep patterns. Frequent interruptions are the norm, whether to check vital signs or assess patients whose conditions are considered unstable. A roommate who is confused or a night owl with the TV blaring is a guarantee of sleep disruption. Sometimes patients report being awakened to ask if they need sleep medication! Lack of sleep is just one more stressor.

Rather than provide a sleeping pill, in my practice, we ask the nursing staff to limit interruptions and use simple relaxation interventions to ease the patient to sleep. Limiting light exposure is also crucial. An important consequence of both cancer and its treatment is fatigue. In many cases, improving sleep will substantially improve this problem. Remarkably few patients with chronic fatigue realize the role their disrupted sleep patterns play in this daytime drowsiness. At home, patients undergoing chemotherapy or radiation may have pain, digestive problems, or other side effects that can disrupt sleep and all of this must be considered along with treatment.

How the Biological Clock Works

We understand the concerns of young professional women who worry that their biological clock is running down on the years remaining to have children. But your biological clock runs on a daily basis. This is known as the circadian rhythm. Normally, your body is alert in the morning and winds down until nighttime, when it is in a natural state to sleep. Before you wake up each day your body temperature and blood pressure rise. Your heart beats faster and your endocrine glands squirt out cortisol and other hormones you need to get going. Then, at night before you go to sleep, temperature, heart rate, and blood pressure fall, and the body releases more melatonin from the base of the brain in response to declining levels of light. Thus, cortisol is active during the day and melatonin is active at night.

Not everybody is a clock watcher, however. Some people naturally get up early and function best during the day, while others tend to come alive at night—or at least they think they do. They may feel happy about it, but their bodies may not agree. Women who work night shifts, for example, are more vulnerable to both breast and colon cancer. Fatigue and loss of appetite are also caused by the skewed circadian rhythm.

The circadian rhythm is part of each cell in your body and in cancer cells the rhythm is out of sync with healthy cells. Cancer can alter circadian function. Thus, the outcome of chemotherapy may reflect differences in circadian rhythms.

Studies have shown that using drugs in morning or evening can make a difference in effectiveness as well as how severe the side effects are. Drugs seem less severe when they are given at the right time. More studies are in progress to learn how the circadian rhythm affects the effectiveness of cancer treatment.

Melatonin: the Night Hormone

The pineal gland produces melatonin. (Artificial melatonin has become popular as a sleep aid and for jet lag.) It is, in fact, a crucial hormone secreted in the early evening as daylight diminishes. This, in turn, triggers a number of physiological responses including an increase in drowsiness, lulling us into a restful sleep. Who has not experienced the sense of sleepiness while on a camping trip, shortly after finishing a fireside dinner and chat, often hours before our usual bedtime? While we often blame this on vigorous hiking and activity, it more likely reflects the burst of melatonin brought on by twilight uninterrupted by the usual artificial light inside our homes.

Melatonin may also be linked to a lower cancer risk, particularly for breast cancer. Women with diminishing eyesight have higher melatonin levels and seem to have a reduced risk of breast cancer, possibly because less light enters their eyes. In animal studies, light interruption at night led to a suppression of their melatonin surge and they had a more rapid tumor growth rate. Adding artificial melatonin reverses this effect. In several breast and prostate cancer studies, melatonin inhibited tumor growth and enhanced the ability of both hormone and chemotherapy to stop tumor cell proliferation. With a disrupted circadian rhythm, the body produces less melatonin and the cell's DNA may be more prone to cancer-causing mutations. We are currently embarking on a study of melatonin in men with prostate cancer who have not responded to both hormonal and chemotherapy treatments. Preliminary data in some patients suggest a significant improvement with the use of melatonin.

Melatonin also slows down the production of estrogen, a hormone that spurs cancerous cells to continue dividing in women with breast and gynecological cancers. Shift workers who work through the night produce less melatonin. As a result, they may produce more cancer-activating estrogen. A study using melatonin in prostate cancer patients revealed a drop of PSA in those who took the drug. Studies in this area are brand-new so we don't have much long-term information yet. However, we do know that a good night's sleep turns on your own melatonin. In addition, melatonin also works as an antioxidant to mop up damaging free radicals while you sleep.

I recommend that my patients who have difficulty sleeping take 3 to 6 milligrams of melatonin around 8 or 9 P.M.

Night Workers and Cancer Risk

In the Harvard Nurses Health Study, a moderate increase in breast cancer was noted in women who worked on rotating night shifts, with at least three nights per month. This risk increased for nurses working over thirty years on night shifts. In a similar study in Seattle, breast cancer risk increased among women who worked the graveyard shift (midnight to 8 A.M.) with risk increasing according to number of years and hours per week.

Women who worked the night shift for fifteen or more years were also at an increased risk for colorectal cancer. As researchers from the Harvard Medical School have suggested, the light is the major factor in resetting the body clock and is reflected in the melatonin secretion pattern, rising with decline of light at night.

Women sleeping in the brightest bedrooms at night appeared to be at some increased risk also. This effect may not be limited to breast cancer, as suggested by a follow-up study from the Nurses Health Study published in 2003.

The known effects of melatonin on cancer cells and the evidence that shift work at night is to blame for increasing cancer risk suggest the role of melatonin as a potential way to protect from cancer. (It also raises questions about the role of nighttime light in the modern world and its impact on increasing cancer risks.)

Cortisol: The Daylight Hormone

When you can't sleep, you feel stressed. This increases production of cortisol, the stress hormone, at a time when melatonin, the sleep hormone, should be working. In a study from Stanford University, sleep problems in ninety-seven women with metastatic breast cancer were evaluated in relation to depression, social support, and cortisol levels. Most women had one or more types of sleep disturbance. More than a third used sleeping pills. Here's what the study found:

* Problems with falling asleep were significantly related to greater pain and depressive symptoms.
* Problems of waking during the night were associated with greater depression and less education.
* Problems in waking and getting up were associated with greater depressive symptoms and less social support.
* Fewer hours of sleep were associated with metastases to the bone and higher depressive symptoms.
* Use of sleeping pills was more frequent among women reporting greater pain and depressive symptoms.
* Women who reported sleeping nine or more hours per night, compared to those who reported six to eight hours, had significantly lower cortisol levels.

These results suggest that the women at higher risk for sleeping problems are depressed, in pain, had cancer spread to the bone, are less educated, or lack social support. Greater quality of social support coincides with lower cortisol concentrations in women with metastatic breast cancer. This indicates healthier neuroendocrine functioning and consequent lower risk for secondary insulin resistance.

Cortisol normally reaches peak levels at dawn then declines throughout the day. People at high risk of breast cancer have a shifted cortisol rhythm. This suggests that when the cortisol cycle is thrown off by troubled sleep, you may also be more cancer prone. Women whose cortisol cycle was shifted also tended to sleep poorly, have lost a spouse or partner, and have cancer-fighting branches of the immune system suppressed. This altered cortisol pattern is also a typical response to severe and prolonged stress.

One of my patients is a perfect example of this. Amanda was forty-five when her husband died. A few months later her house burned down. Then within the year she was diagnosed with an aggressive breast cancer. She had also gained a good deal of weight during this stressful year, and I suspected even before testing her that she wasn't sleeping well, and she was churning out lots of cortisol because of all the stress. Fortunately, we brought this under control with a variety of medications and interventional care.

Overcoming a Common Problem: Some Sleep Techniques

Now you know why you need a good night's sleep and why inadequate sleep is one of the most common problems for cancer patients. The normal sleep cycle is integral to maintaining normal hormone levels. And that is crucial in making cancer treatment most effective.

If you have problems sleeping during your cancer therapy, talk with your doctor about medication that may help you. You may need sleeping pills for the short term. In addition, there are many things you can do yourself. I ask my patients with sleep problems to keep a diary and try to pinpoint the hours before sleep and what occurs. Then we can try to figure out what might be keeping them awake and what we can do to change that situation. The mind-body techniques in chapter 12 can also help you sleep better.

Stretching and Exercise

Don't exercise too close to bedtime because exercise acts as a stimulant. Instead, exercise regularly four to six hours before bedtime. The benefit of moderate-intensity activity on sleep quality depends on the amount of exercise and the time of day it is performed. A new study in October 2003 from the American Academy of Sleep Medicine found that stretching and exercise may improve sleep quality in overweight, postmenopausal women. The new findings were revealed by researchers at Seattle's Fred Hutchinson Cancer Research Center. Women who exercised at moderate intensity for at least half an hour each morning, seven days a week, had less trouble falling asleep than those who exercised less. Conversely, women who performed evening exercises experienced little or no improvement in sleep onset or quality. One possible explanation is that morning versus evening exercise may change the circadian rhythm that affects sleep quality.

Eating and Drinking

Eat a light snack about an hour before bedtime. A glass of milk increases brain levels of tryptophan, an amino acid in protein that will help you sleep. Tryptophan increases your body's production of melatonin and serotonin.

For three to six hours before bedtime avoid alcohol, spicy foods and greasy and heavy foods that are hard to digest. Naturally, you should avoid caffeine in the latter part of the day. And this means not only the caffeine in coffee, but in tea, soft drinks, or chocolate. My patients with chemotherapy-induced chocolate cravings have told me of having a cup of hot chocolate before bed. If it's made with milk, you increase the level of tryptophan to aid sleep, but the chocolate is full of caffeine. Coffee ice cream or yogurt, by the way, contains enough caffeine to keep you awake.

Create a Routine

Get into a routine for bedtime and keep regular sleep hours, especially for waking up. Relax in the evening as bedtime approaches. Just by beginning a bedtime ritual your body and mind get signals that it's time to sleep. Sometimes a warm bath will relax you, especially if you precede or follow it with some mind-body techniques. Imagine yourself enjoying a sound sleep. Think of how warm and comforting your bed feels. Imagine the soothing feel of soft sheets against your skin.

Reading and watching television in bed are two popular end-of-day activities. One man told me he liked to watch TV at night, so he went into the living room where they had a TV. His wife didn't want a TV in the bedroom but liked to read in bed. Each night, when the man went to bed he found his wife asleep. He removed her eyeglasses, closed her book, and turned out the light. On the other hand, many people use TV as a sleeping pill and have an automatic timer on the set in the bedroom. Something about the low drone of the sound (and perhaps the boring nature of the programming) seems to send them right into oblivion. However, in general, using the television as a sleep aid is probably not a good idea. You end up waking up in the middle of the night to turn it off, and the TV also lights up the room, which may inhibit sleep.

Set the Mood

Keep the bedroom quiet and comfortable, not too hot or cold. Cool is best, as your body temperature and other internal operating systems cool down, too. If your bedroom is in a location that allows bright lights to shine through the windows, then get drapes that can close out the light. On the other hand, you want plenty of light to flood inside in the morning, in sync with your body clock.

Your bedroom should be a serene place with little or no clutter. If your bed is comfortable, make it even more comfortable with the addition of a featherbed on your mattress. This adds a layer of cloudlike softness. Use soft cotton sheets and make sure your pillows are comfortable. The wrong pillows can keep you awake without your knowing it. If you sleep on your stomach, you need soft pillows. If you are a side or back sleeper, the pillows should have some firmness.

If You Don't Succeed, Get Up

Try to go to bed when you are sleepy. However, if you don't fall asleep in twenty minutes, don't stay there. Get up and do something distracting, but not stimulating.

I recommend going into another room and writing down all the things that are going through your mind and preventing sleep. Write down this internal dialogue. By releasing it you put it to rest—and then you can get some rest yourself.

You don't want to worry about sleep or tomorrow. If you lie in bed worrying about not being able to sleep, you become stressed and cortisol pumps up and wakes you up even more.

Cancer Treatment by the Clock:
A Future Possibility

Chronotherapy is a type of therapy that considers the patient's circadian rhythm during treatment for illness, including cancer. So far it is experimental but studies with animals show that giving chemotherapy at specific stages of the rest and activity cycle improves the effectiveness of the treatment and reduces the side effects of chemotherapy. This has been used in both colon and ovarian cancer.

A study of colon cancer found that peak delivery time for chemo was 4 A.M. We can't wake you up at home, but special ways of delivering chemotherapy through a pump while you are asleep can be achieved. Hopefully, ongoing studies will show us practical and effective ways of using this in cancer treatment.

We do know how to check a person's circadian rhythm with actigraphy. This involves wearing a small wrist piezoelectric accelerometer. Patients in a study wore it for three consecutive twenty-four-hour spans. Each patient kept a diary for times of rising and retiring. By measuring the rest and activity cycle as a major circadian clock output, actigraphy provides a simple tool for evaluating cancer patients. Circadian rhythms can also be checked with blood tests to look at cortisol and white blood cell counts collected at different times of day.

THE DAMAGING biology of stress continues while you sleep— or don't sleep. Managing stress responses by adopting healthy eating and exercise habits, getting a good night's sleep, and finding good emotional and social support should be regarded as much a part of cancer treatment as chemotherapy or radiation. Doctors should not just fight the tumor, but help the people with the disease to live with it.

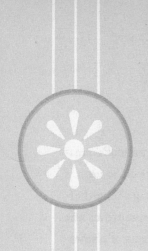

CHAPTER 15

Follow-up Care: Don't Fall off the Cliff

YOUR LAST CHEMOTHERAPY or radiation treatment is technically called the end of treatment. At the end of radiation, chemotherapy, or surgery, doctors and the other health-care providers encourage you to celebrate. Your doctor will tell you there is no evidence of disease, but you need to come in for checkups so you can be watched closely for the next few months. But after the close monitoring and almost daily contact and visits, it feels like being dropped off a cliff to patients and their family members. As a cancer patient, you felt the busy schedule and regular support of nurses and doctors had a supportive psychological and medical value.

Even though they are glad the procedures are completed, many patients say they feel depressed and anxious when their treatment ends, sometimes more than they felt during treatment. These emotions, which may have been evident intermittently throughout treatment, may emerge immediately after treatment or may even appear six to nine months after active treatment ends.

I have heard patients say, "I felt so strong then, and now I feel weak and vulnerable." Or, "I was so busy with the rigors of treatment that I didn't have time to think about what was really happening to me . . . now what?"

Confronting the emotions, the changes, and the lifelong concerns resulting from cancer may be delayed during treatment. You had a busy appointment schedule. You had to cope with side effects. Your medical team was always around. In addition to this falloff in contact with the medical team, your family and friends may seem scarce now that you are okay and back to normal. You may feel you've been deserted by everyone.

The technique of focusing on the tiny details to avoid the looming and frightening larger threat was easier during treatment. When these distractions disappear, you are left to wage a private inner battle with your doubts, fears, and life changes.

You may wonder if your feelings of depression, anxiety, fear, and sadness are normal and if your worries, uncertainties, and fears are valid. High levels of anxiety and worry about unknown factors are common at the beginning *and end of treatment*. It is important to acknowledge them. You may feel helpless and hopeless. There is a very natural fear of the cancer's recurrence, residual fatigue, self-doubt, and poor self-image.

When my patients complete their treatment I assure them that I am not abandoning them. I am changing the focus and frequency of their visits. I explain the follow-up treatment and I encourage them to call us with any concerns they have. I would never brush off anyone with a casual wave of the hand saying, "Oh, you'll be fine." I have heard of doctors who made their patients feel guilty by asking them, "How could you feel this way after we fought so hard to save your life?"

Accept none of these comments. In our medical system you

need to be sure you get the right kind of follow-up care, not just to monitor your cancer, but for prevention and treatment of all the other medical conditions that can occur. Once you survive cancer you are part of a vulnerable patient population because your cancer diagnosis shifts attention away from important noncancer problems. Doctors need to be alerted to this so you receive good care.

Medicare claims of 14,884 survivors of colorectal cancer were analyzed in a study. There was an increased likelihood of cancer survivors compared with the general public in not receiving recommended care across a broad range of chronic medical conditions. They were not likely to get care from both primary-care and oncology doctors. African Americans and the elderly were even less likely to get what they needed.

A possible explanation is that patients lose contact with noncancer providers who are important to their care. If your primary-care physician was not involved in your cancer treatment, it decreases your likelihood of receiving appropriate health maintenance.

Stay in touch with your primary-care physician, even if that person is one of the specialists you use. Know the role that doctor plays in your care and be sure that you get recommendations both for cancer surveillance and routine preventive health. Be sure that all of your doctors know your health history. This may affect their treatment for other conditions.

Keep your own medical records up to date. Each time you have a checkup, make a note of what occurred and when the next checkup is due. Mark it on your calendar. Most of my patients have put their own medical records on their computer system so they can easily update them.

Cancer Survivors Program

For all the above reasons, it is necessary to be part of a cancer survivors program and today we have such programs. The National Cancer Institute for Cancer Survivorship (www.survivorship. cancer.gov) recently published a report called *Living Beyond Cancer: Finding a New Balance.* This report provides information about preventing a recurrence of cancer and confirms that cancer survivors tend to be underscreened after their treatment ends—not only for recurrent cancer, but for all other conditions as well. The report is available on their Web site. You can also find regional "Live Strong" groups that are designed to help cancer survivors get the proper screening and health care.

Other resources for cancer survivors include:

* The National Coalition for Cancer Survivors at www. canceradvocacy.org
* The Association of Cancer Online Resources at www.acor.org
* The Annie Appleseed Project at www.annieappleseed.com

Monitoring Good Health

Once you have been treated for cancer, you will want to maintain a schedule of follow-up care, such as blood tests, mammograms, PSAs, and other surveillance, for the rest of your life. After cancer treatment, you must have follow-up visits with your oncology doctor every few months during the first year. In addition, you need to do the following:

* Check for metabolic syndrome. We check our patients every two months during treatment and continue that practice af-

ter treatment ends. After the first two checkups, we check every six months and then annually.

✳ Have blood tests for cancer markers as well as inflammation. These should be done every three months for the first two years, then twice a year for three years, then annually.

✳ Regular preventive checkups should include an annual mammogram (possibly more after breast cancer), colonoscopy, and other tests, depending upon your condition. If you have had one cancer, you may be more vulnerable to another. For example, some doctors want their breast cancer patients to get a colonoscopy every two or three years rather than the usual five years.

And while you will no longer be receiving chemotherapy, radiation, or other treatment for the cancer, you should always keep up the new ways of eating, physical activity, and stress control. This will help you prevent a recurrence or new cancer, and it will be good for your entire family, too.

Many survivors find cancer a wake-up call to get rid of bad habits, especially smoking. They learn to eat better and get off the couch more often. Reducing stress may be more difficult, but many succeed.

Millions of people have survived cancer and remain free of it, often after prolonged and high-dose chemotherapy and radiation. Many have survived the rigors of bone-marrow transplantation. Despite the ominous implications of cancer diagnosis, this legion of heroic people testifies to the benefits of the best conventional medical care as well as to the emotional strength of patients and their families and friends, sustaining them through this fight.

Stick to all of the lessons you've learned in this book about nutrition, exercise, and stress reduction—and have a good, long life.

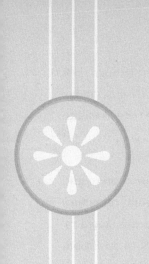

Leaving a Healthy Legacy for Our Children

INSULIN RESISTANCE OFTEN BEGINS in childhood. The causes of the metabolic syndrome include progressive weight gain during early adolescence through adulthood, inadequate physical activity (not simply in exercise but generalized decrease in energy expenditure typical of modern lifestyles), and more recently the presence of chronic stress.

Body weight along with blood pressure among school-age children has increased progressively over the past decade. There is also evidence of blood vessel changes in obese children. Fatty plaques have been discovered in the coronary arteries of children dying in adolescence.

Not only are children fatter, they are starting to develop real disease—type 2 diabetes is increasing among children. Abnormal glucose tolerance is frequently seen among overweight children and we may need to begin performing routine glucose tolerance tests on children. Studies show a strong correlation in body mass index (BMI) at ages eight, thirteen, and twenty-five, so parents need to concern themselves with overweight children and not shrug it off as baby fat that they will outgrow.

Recent research also indicates that undernutrition in utero and in the first year of life also increases the risk of insulin resistance and glucose intolerance in early adulthood. It is accompanied by rapid weight gain in adolescence. Again, it goes back to evolution. If a fetus is constantly deprived of calories during prenatal development, the presumption is its metabolic state will be permanently altered to enhance energy storage (fat production), like a mini-version of the thrifty phenotype. When food is around, they will more aggressively produce body fat.

Familial influences are also very important. There is significant correlation between parents and children in both weight and insulin sensitivity. Puberty is associated with insulin resistance, and body size changes dramatically, with greater increase in body fat in girls and lean body mass in boys. Boys show a decrease in insulin sensitivity during adolescence.

In a study by Alan Sinaiko, a pediatric professor at the University of Minnesota, reported at the first World Congress on the Insulin Resistance Syndrome, and published in *Diabetes Care,* March 2004, the prevalence of metabolic syndrome was 2, 4, and 8 percent at ages thirteen, fifteen, and nineteen. He suggested that these criteria may underestimate the prevalence of IR among children.

Susan, a middle-aged homemaker, learned to understand the risk her own children faced after her bout with cancer. She came to me after being diagnosed with colon cancer that had not yet spread beyond the colon wall. She had been slightly overweight during late childhood and adolescence but her weight had skyrocketed after the birth of her three children. At the time of her initial visit she weighed 160 pounds and was forty pounds overweight. She was only five feet three, leaving her with a body mass index between 28 and 29, and her waist measured thirty-eight inches. Unlike many women her age, Susan's fat was mostly distributed toward her midsection and not her hips. Because of her busy and hectic schedule with three active adolescent kids, she found little time for her own needs.

Further tests confirmed that Susan had the metabolic syndrome and after taking a careful history, it became apparent she was not alone in the family. Her father and paternal aunt had both developed diabetes in their late fifties and her father had pancreatic cancer at sixty-four and died a year later. One of her three sisters had breast cancer at fifty-four and was now well, but also overweight. Also of concern, two of Susan's children were significantly overweight.

After surgery, Susan had chemotherapy. In light of strong evidence for the metabolic syndrome, a program of diet and progressive exercise was outlined, with particular attention paid to coordinating this with her ongoing chemotherapy. Most important, we also convinced her to get her kids involved in a program of nutrition and exercise.

The Diabetes-Cancer Link

Seventeen million Americans have diabetes. More than 90 percent have type 2 and upward of a third of these are unaware of having this disorder and its potentially serious consequences. Another sixteen million or more have a condition called prediabetes, which is a harbinger for the eventual development of type 2 diabetes, or noninsulin-dependent diabetes. This subgroup, in fact, represents those members of the population who are overweight and who indeed have an insulin-resistant state in the metabolic syndrome. Worldwide, 194 million people have diabetes and the number is growing dramatically along with the obesity epidemic in developing nations as they adopt Western lifestyles.

Even more disturbing is a new estimate of a lifetime risk of developing diabetes among children who are born in the year 2000. An analysis published in 2003 in the *Journal of the American Medical Association* by scientists at the Centers for Disease Control and Prevention predicts that, of children born in the year 2000, more than a third of whites, two in five blacks, and half of Hispanics are destined to be diabetic unless drastic lifestyle changes are made.

Well before diabetes develops, many people, particularly those with significant abdominal obesity, will develop signs of the metabolic syndrome accompanied by abnormal lipids, impaired glucose tolerance, and evidence of insulin resistance with high circulating insulin levels. This longstanding high insulin level sets the stage for the development of cancers such as pancreatic carcinoma. The link between obesity and breast cancer and other hormonal cancers, as already noted, has in part been explained by the impact of obesity on higher levels of estrogen and other important hormones that stimulate these hormone-sensitive tumors. However, the same relationship with obesity applies to nonhormone-sensitive cancers such as pancreatic, colon, and esophageal. The links between obesity, insulin, and pancreatic cancer are becoming well documented.

Pancreatic tumor cells have higher levels of insulin as well as IGF type 1 receptors than normal cells. As cancers progress, these receptors are activated by circulating insulin and IGF-1. Animal studies have shown that rising insulin levels lead to a higher cancer risk and that when exercise levels are raised, insulin levels drop and less cancer results.

As noted in the *Journal of the American Medical Association* study of adults who were obese and had a high risk for pancreatic cancer, the role of chronic insulin production is likely the crucial link between the risk for pancreatic cancer and obesity via the metabolic syndrome and the accompanying insulin-resistant state.

In an American Cancer Society study, a history of diabetes was significantly related to death from pancreatic cancer in both men and women, even when they had diabetes for many years before getting cancer. The National Cancer Institute has studied pancreatic cancer in the United States and found a significant positive trend with increasing number of years of diabetes preceding the pancreatic cancer diagnosis. If you have had diabetes for at least ten years you have a 50 percent greater risk of pancreatic cancer.

In a study of people in the Chicago area, those with insulin resistance, particularly men, had a significant increase in pancreatic cancer risk. Women who had diets of highly refined carbohydrates had a 53 percent increase in risk. This trend is most apparent in women who are overweight with a high body mass index and low levels of physical activity. Combined, that risk is 267 percent—again linking diet, exercise, and an insulin-resistant state to this disease. These studies turn our previous understanding of pancreatic cancer on its head. Because of its effect on the cells producing insulin, we had assumed that the cancer itself, by reducing the ability of the pancreas to produce insulin, might indeed be a cause of diabetes. We now believe that diabetes may actually be an important cause of pancreatic cancer.

Diabetes is a disorder of blood sugar regulation. In both type 1 and type 2 diabetes, glucose builds up in the blood to serious levels, spills into the urine, and causes increased thirst and frequency of urination. Specialized cells in the pancreas—islet cells—produce the insulin that assists in transporting glucose from the blood into the cells. It is then used for energy or it can be converted into metabolites that are available to store for future energy use or eventually channeled into fat storage. This means it is changed to production of adipose fatty acids and triglycerides for fat stores.

In type 1 diabetes, a form of autoimmune disease, these cells fail to produce enough insulin. However, in type 2, or noninsulin-dependent diabetes, which is rising in direct proportion to the level of obesity in the population, the body typically produces enough insulin at first to maintain blood sugar control. The cells in the muscles and fat become increasingly resistant to the action of insulin. As a result, blood sugar levels rise so the pancreas is forced to secrete higher and higher levels of insulin to maintain relative blood sugar control. Eventually, the pancreatic cells are incapable of maintaining adequate insulin output and eventually diabetes develops with accompanying insulin insufficiency.

How Diabetes Causes Pancreatic Cancer

Peter, a retired executive, gained weight gradually during middle age until he had a BMI of 34 and a waist of forty-two inches. In his early sixties, he developed an unexplained increase in numbness and tingling in his feet that led to difficulty with walking on occasion. Several years later, just prior to seeing me, he developed increasing abdominal pain and his internist ordered a CT scan, which revealed a large pancreatic mass and lesions within his liver. A CT-guided biopsy of the pancreas confirmed cancer.

Peter's triglycerides were 240, his fasting insulin level was 24, his fasting blood sugar was 112, and he had low HDL cholesterol. Although not yet diabetic, Peter had clear-cut evidence for the metabolic syndrome. After careful discussion with him, we put Peter on a diet and exercise regimen to try to correct his metabolic abnormalities. At the same time he began conventional chemotherapy with gemcitabine and a low dose of another medicine. Within six months his pancreatic tumor mass had disappeared and there were minimally visible lesions within the liver. Peter also lost fifteen pounds and had normalized his insulin and lipid levels. Over the next six months he continued to do well in maintaining his regimen.

One year after Peter's initial diagnosis, repeat scans suggested an increase in his lesions and his metabolic studies indicated a bump in his insulin level and his triglycerides, consistent with worsening signs of the metabolic syndrome. He was then restarted on a more aggressive dietary regimen and he also restarted his original chemotherapy medication. Rather than switch to a different medicine, which is typical in cancer treatment, we decided to use the same medication again. Once again, Peter had a profound reduction in tumor size and has for two and a half years remained free of disease. This illustrates that insulin may play a role, not only in causing pancreatic cancer, but in the effectiveness of chemotherapy for this disease, known to be very resistant to conventional chemotherapy.

A single patient does not prove this relationship, but it shows a profoundly important relationship. Very often, patients are assumed to be resistant to chemotherapy and alternative medicines are used at the time of progression. In this case, however, the key intervening feature was recurrence of signs of insulin resistance, which was treated aggressively, and subsequent retreatment with the same medicines showed a dramatic response and now significant long-term survival with minimal evidence of pancreatic cancer progression.

The proof is all around us and it is overwhelming, not only for ourselves, but for our children and grandchildren. The stories of people in this book illustrate the importance of much needed reform in our lifestyles. The triad of poor diet, lack of physical activity, and increasing stress has set us up for a shorter life at a time in history when it should be extended. We need to encourage a triad of good nutrition, physical activity, and reduction of stress. Then, hopefully, we can prevent much of the cancer that strikes so many.

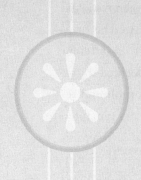

Cancer Information Resources

American Cancer Society
1-800-ACS-2345 (1-800-227-2345)
http://www.cancer.org

With 3,400 chapters in the United States, this is the largest voluntary health agency in the world. ACS sponsors research, education, and patient service programs, including transportation to and from treatment, support groups, and equipment loans. It is usually a good way to find out what resources are available in your community.

American College of Surgeons Commission on Cancer
633 N. St. Clair Street
Chicago, IL 60611
http://www.facs.org/cancer/coc/coc.html

Write for a booklet listing approved cancer programs. Revised quarterly.

American Society of Clinical Oncology
www.asco.org

This is a professional organization of doctors who treat cancer. ASCO has more than 21,500 members in over one hundred countries. Members specialize in all fields of oncology, including medical, hematology, therapeutic radiology, surgery, and pediatric care. They can help you locate a doctor in your area.

American Society for Therapeutic Radiology and Oncology
12500 Fair Lakes Circle, Suite 375
Fairfax, VA 22033-3382
Phone: 703-502-1550 or 800-962-7876
Fax: 703-502-7852
www.astro.org

This is the professional organization of radiation oncologists. They can help you locate one in your area.

Breast Cancer Alliance
Box 414
15 East Putnam Avenue
Greenwich, CT 06830
203-861-0014
info@breastcancer.org

The Breast Cancer Alliance funds innovative breast cancer research and promotes breast health through education and outreach. It is expanding its role as the preeminent regional organization funding breast cancer research, early detection, and education.

Cancer Care

http://www.cancercare.org

Web site of the oldest (1944) and largest national nonprofit agency providing emotional support, information, and practical help to people with cancer and their loved ones.

CancerLinks

http://www.cancerlinks.org

Site designed to make searching the World Wide Web for information about cancer faster and easier.

CancerLinksUSA

http://www.cancerlinksusa.com

Noncommercial site founded to provide support and information to cancer patients and their caregivers.

Corporate Angel Network (CAN)

http://www.corpangelnetwork.org

This organization provides cancer patients with free air transportation to and from medical facilities using empty seats on corporate aircraft. Patients must meet CAN's qualifications, but they don't need to meet any financial-need criteria.

The Chemotherapy Foundation

183 Madison Avenue

New York, NY 10016

Phone: 1-212-213-9292

Ask for their free forty-page booklet on chemotherapy. It explains in detail how chemotherapy works, which drugs are used, and more.

International Union Against Cancer
www.uicc.org

This is the largest independent, nonprofit, nongovernmental association of 280 cancer organizations in over eighty countries. It is a global resource for action and voice and brings together individuals including advocacy groups, patients, survivor support groups, public health authorities, and research and treatment centers.

Memorial Sloan-Kettering Cancer Center
http://www.mskcc.org

Web site of the world's oldest and largest private institution (established in 1884) devoted to prevention, patient care, research, and education in cancer.

M. D. Anderson Cancer Center, University of Texas
http://www.mdanderson.org

Web site of one of the National Cancer Institute's designated Comprehensive Cancer Centers focused exclusively on cancer patient care, research, education, and prevention.

NCI Cancer Information Service Hotline
1-800-4-CANCER (1-800-422-6237)

The National Cancer Institute (NCI) is the primary federal agency for cancer research and information on everything from clinical trials to new drugs. The hotline is operated by a network of authorized comprehensive cancer centers, and you will be connected with the one nearest you. NCI keeps an up-to-date file of available resources and physicians. The hotline operates weekdays from 9 A.M. to 4:30 P.M. eastern standard time.

Material is from PDQ, a computer service that gives up-to-date information on cancer treatment. It is a service for people with cancer and their families and for doctors, nurses, and other health-care professionals. PDQ information is reviewed each month by cancer experts and is updated when the information changes. PDQ also lists information about research on new treatments, clinical trials, doctors who treat cancer, and hospitals with cancer programs.

You can obtain information from NCI by fax or through the Internet.

CancerFax
301-402-5874

CancerFax is a way to obtain PDQ information statements in English or Spanish using a fax machine. It contains fact sheets on various cancer topics from NCI's office of cancer communications. CancerFax operates twenty-four hours a day, seven days a week, with no other charge than the telephone call. For a fact sheet explaining how to use CancerFax, call 1-800-4-CANCER.

CancerNet
cancernet@icicc.nci.nih.gov

Enter the word HELP in the body of the mail message. The information is also available in Spanish. CancerNet will send you a return mail message containing the contents list of materials available through the CancerNet.

Cancer Trials
http://www.cancer.gov/clinicaltrials

Comprehensive clinical trial information for patients, health-care professionals, and the public.

National Coalition for Cancer Survivorship (NCCS)
1010 Wayne Avenue, Suite 300
Silver Spring, MD 20910
Phone: 301-585-2616
www.canceradvocacy.org

This network of independent groups and individuals is concerned with support of cancer survivors and their families. NCCS's primary goal is to promote a national awareness of issues affecting cancer survivors. Its objectives are to serve as a clearinghouse for information on services and materials for survivors, advocate their rights and interests, encourage the study of survivorship, and promote the development of cancer support activities.

OncoLink of the University of Pennsylvania
http://cancer.med.upenn.edu

Founded in 1994 by Penn cancer specialists with a mission to help cancer patients, families, health-care professionals, and the general public get accurate cancer-related information at no charge.

Society for Integrative Oncology
19 Mantua Road
Mount Royal, NJ 08061
Phone: 856-423-7222
Fax: 856-423-3420
www.integrativeonc.org
Email: siohq@tally.com

This is a nonprofit, multidisciplinary organization dedicated to studying and facilitating the cancer treatment and recovery process through the use of integrated complementary therapies. Their mission is to educate oncology professionals, patients, caregivers, and relevant others about state-of-the art integrative therapies, including their scientific validity, clinical benefits, toxicities, and limitations.

The Susan G. Komen Breast Cancer Foundation
www.komen.org

This group sponsors a twenty-four-hour toll-free hotline for information: 1-800-I'M AWARE (1-800-462-9273).

U.S. Department of Health and Human Services and the
U.S. Department of Agriculture
http://www.health.gov/dietaryguidelines/dga2005/report

Go to this website for the 2005 dietary guidelines for Americans. These new government guidelines are very similar to those in this book.

Women's Cancer Network
http://www.wcn.org

Site developed by the Gynecologic Cancer Foundation and dedicated to informing women around the world about gynecologic cancer.

Pediatric Cancer Information

The Pediatric Cancer Care Network is a collaboration of two NCI-sponsored cooperative groups that study children's cancers and the Blue Cross and Blue Shield Association. The network's purpose is to ensure that children of Blue Cross and Blue Shield subscribers receive care at designated centers of cancer excellence. The Web sites of Blue Cross and Blue Shield, Candlelighters, National Childhood Cancer Foundation, and Pediatric Oncology Group listed here compose this network.

Candlelighters Childhood Cancer Foundation (CCCF)
www.candlelighters.org

This site is an introduction to the programs and services of CCCF, including publications and local chapters. CCCF is an international nonprofit organization dedicated to educating, supporting, serving, and advocating for families of children with cancer, survivors of childhood cancer, and the professionals who care for them.

Children's Cancer Research Fund
www.ccrf-kids.org

Its goal is to establish and foster research in childhood cancer, as well as enrich the quality of life for children with cancer by improving clinical and support services.

National Childhood Cancer Foundation/Children's Oncology Group (NCCF/COG)
www.curesearch.org

Information about the facts of childhood cancer, stories of cancer survivors, clinical trial information of Children's Cancer Group, and locations of CCG institutions. A separate password-protected area is maintained for CCG membership. This area contains detailed CCG protocols, group-operational information, and group collaboration services such as group-specific mailing lists and Web-based conference board.

Books

Benson, Herbert. *The Relaxation Response*. New York: Harper-Torch, 1976.

Dreher, Henry. *Mind-Body Unity: A New Vision for Mind-Body Science and Medicine*. Baltimore: Johns Hopkins Press, 2004.

Huddleston, Peggy. *Prepare for Surgery, Heal Faster: A Guide of Mind-Body Techniques*. Angel River Press, 1996.

Kabat-Zinn, John. *Full Catastrophe Living: Using the Wisdom of Your Body and Mind to Face Stress, Pain, and Illness*. New York: Delta, 1990.

Khalsa, Gurucharan Singh, and Yogi Bhajan. *BreathWalk: Breathing Your Way to a Revitalized Body, Mind, and Spirit*. New York: Broadway Books, 2000.

Lerner, Michael. *Choices in Healing: Integrating the Best of Conventional and Complementary Approaches to Cancer*. Cambridge: MIT Press, 1996.

Nixon, Daniel. *Cancer Recovery Eating Plan: The Right Foods to Help Fuel Your Recovery*. New York: Three Rivers Press, 1996.

Tagliaferri, Mary, Isaac Cohen, and Debu Tripathy, eds. *Breast Cancer: Beyond Convention—The World's Foremost Authorities on Complementary and Alternative Medicine Offer Advice on Healing*. New York: Atria Books, 2002.

Selected Journal References

Albert, D. S., M. E. Martinez, D. J. Roe, et al. "Lack of Effect of a High Fiber Cereal Supplement on the Recurrence of Colorectal Adenomas." *New England Journal of Medicine*, no. 342 (2000): 1156–62.

Amling, C. L., C. J. Kane, and R. H. Riffensburgh. "Relationship Between Obesity and Race in Predicting Adverse Pathologic Variables in Patients Undergoing Radical Prostatectomy." *Urology* 58, no. 5 (2001): 723–28.

Balkwill, F., and A. Mantovani. "Inflammation and Cancer: Back to Virchow?" *Lancet* 357, no. 9255 (2001): 539–45.

Block, K. I., D. B. Boyd, N. Gonzalez, and A. Vojdani. "Point Counterpoint: The Immune System in Cancer Integrative Therapies." *Integrative Cancer Therapies* 2, no. 4 (2003): 315–29.

Boyd, D. B. "Insulin and Cancer." *Integrative Cancer Therapies* 2, no. 4 (2003): 315–29.

Bruce, W. R., T. M. Wolever, and A. Giacca. "Mechanisms Linking Diet and Colorectal Cancer: The Possible Role of Insulin Resistance." *Nutrition and Cancer* 37, no. 1 (2000): 19–26.

Byers, T. "Nutritional Risk Factors for Breast Cancer." *Cancer* 74 (1994): S288–S295.

Caloe, F. E., C. Rodriquez, K. Walker-Thurmond, and M. J. Thun. "Overweight, Obesity, and Mortality from Cancer in a Prospectively Studied Cohort of U.S. Adults." *New England Journal of Medicine* 348, no. 17 (2003): 1625–1638.

Carroll, K. K. "Obesity as a Risk Factor for Certain Types of Cancer." *Lipids*, no. 33 (1998): 1055–59.

Daling, J., E. K. Malone, D. R. Doody, et al. "Relations of Body Mass Index to Tumor Markers and Survival Among Young Women with Invasive Ductal Breast Carcinomas." *Cancer* 92, no. 4 (2001): 720–29.

Friedenreich, C. M., and J. R. Orenstein. "Physical Activity and Cancer Prevention: Etiologic Evidence and Biological Mechanisms." *Journal of Nutrition* 132, Suppl. no. 11 (2002): 34565–34645.

Goodwin, P. J., M. Ennis, K. I. Pritchard, et al. "Fasting Insulin and Outcome in Early-Stage Breast Cancer: Results of Prospective Cohort Study." *Journal of Clinical Oncology* 20, no. 1 (2002): 42–51.

Huntington, M. O. "Weight Gain in Patients Receiving Adjuvant Chemotherapy for Carcinoma of the Breast." *Cancer* 56, no. 3 (1985): 472–74.

McMillan, D. C., K. Canna, and C. S. McArdle. "Measurement of the Systemic Inflammatory Response Predicts Cancer Specific and Non-Cancer Survival in Patients with Cancer." *Nutrition and Cancer* 41, nos. 1–2 (2001): 64–69.

Michaud, D. S., E. Giovannucci, W. C. Wilet, et al. "Physical Activity, Obesity, Height, and the Risk of Pancreatic Cancer." *Journal of the American Medical Association* 286, no. 8 (2001): 921–29.

Moschos, S. J., and C. S. Mantozoros. "The Role of the IGF System in Cancer: From Basic to Clinical Studies and Clinical Applications." *Oncology* 65, no. 4 (2002): 317–22.

Rosmond, R. "Stress Induced Disturbances of the HPA Axis: A Pathway to Type 2 Diabetes?" *Medical Science Monthly* 9, no. 2 (2003): RA 35–39.

Sandu, M. S., D. B. Dunger, and E. L. Giovannuci. "Insulin, Insulin-like Growth Factor-1 (IGF-1), IGF-1 Binding Proteins, Their Biological Interactions, and Colorectal Cancer." *Journal of the National Cancer Institute*, no. 94 (2002): 972–80.

Sephton, S. E., R. M. Sapolsky, H. C. Kraemer, et al. "Diurnal Cortisol Rhythm as a Predictor of Breast Cancer Survival." *Journal of the National Cancer Institute* 92, no. 12 (2000): 994–1000.

Spiegel, D., J. R. Bloom, H. C. Kraemer, et al. "Effect of Psychological Treatment on Survival of Patients with Metastatic Breast Cancer." *Lancet* 2, no. 8668 (1989): 888–91.

Watson, M., J. S. Haviland, S. Greer, et al. "Influence of Psychological Response on Survival in Breast Cancer: A Population Based Cohort Study." *Lancet* 354, no. 9187 (1999): 1331–36.

Index

About the Authors

D. BARRY BOYD, MD, is founder and director of the Integrative Medicine Program at Greenwich Hospital—Yale Medical Center. Dr. Boyd teaches medical residents at the Yale Cancer Center and formerly taught at The New York Presbyterian Hospital Weill Cornell Medical Center, where he helped set up the Center for Complementary and Integrative Medicine. He has written many academic papers about integrative cancer care. Dr. Boyd's expertise is frequently sought by the media and cancer support groups, such as Gilda's Club and Man to Man. He lives in Greenwich, Connecticut.

MARIAN BETANCOURT has had breast cancer herself and is the coauthor of several health books, including *What to Do When You Get Breast Cancer* (Little, Brown); *What to Do When You Get Colon Cancer,* and *The Doctor's Guide to Gastrointestinal Health* (Wiley); *The Coming Cancer Breakthroughs* (Kensington); as well as *What's in the Air: The Complete Guide to Airborne Allergies* and *Say Good-bye to Back Pain* (Pocket). She is the author of two books on women's issues and has written hundreds of newspaper and magazine articles. She lives in New York City.